WASH, WEAR, AND CARE

WASH, WEAR, *and* CARE

Clothing and Laundry in Long-Term Residential Care

PAT ARMSTRONG and SUZANNE DAY

McGill-Queen's University Press

Montreal & Kingston · London · Chicago

ISBN 978-0-7735-4922-7 (cloth)
ISBN 978-0-7735-4923-4 (paper)
ISBN 978-0-7735-4924-1 (ePDF)
ISBN 978-0-7735-4925-8 (ePUB)   .

Legal deposit second quarter 2017
Bibliothèque nationale du Québec

Printed in Canada on acid-free paper that is 100% ancient forest free
(100% post-consumer recycled), processed chlorine free.

This book has been published with the help of a grant from the
Canadian Federation for the Humanities and Social Sciences, through
the Awards to Scholarly Publications Program, using funds provided
by the Social Sciences and Humanities Research Council of Canada.

McGill-Queen's University Press acknowledges the support of the
Canada Council for the Arts for our publishing program. We also
acknowledge the financial support of the Government of Canada
through the Canada Book Fund for our publishing activities.

Library and Archives Canada Cataloguing in Publication

Armstrong, Pat, 1945–, author
    Wash, wear, and care : clothing and laundry in long-term residential care
/ Pat Armstrong and Suzanne Day.

Includes bibliographical references and index.
Issued in print and electronic formats.
ISBN 978-0-7735-4922-7 (hardcover). – ISBN 978-0-7735-4923-4 (softcover). –
ISBN 978-0-7735-4924-1 (ePDF). – ISBN 978-0-7735-4925-8 (ePUB)

    1. Nursing home patients – Clothing – Social aspects. 2. Nursing home
patients – Clothing – Psychological aspects. 3. Laundry – Social aspects.
4. Autonomy (Psychology) in old age. 5. Older people – Health and hygiene.
6. Older people – Long-term care. 7. Textbooks. I. Day, Suzanne, 1982–,
author II. Title.

RA999.S36A76 2017   362.6'1   C2016-907638-5
                                                 C2016-907639-3

This book was typeset by True to Type in 10.5/13 Sabon

Contents

Acknowledgments

On behalf of the entire team, we would like to thank the long-term residential care homes and all those who work and live within them for sharing so much with us. We have been impressed with the dedication and commitment of those who provide care and of those who manage care, as well as with the strength of the residents and their families. While we identified problems, we also saw many ideas worth sharing. On behalf of Pat and Suzanne, we would like to thank all those who participated in the ethnographic work. Their skilled observations and interviews constitute the primary data for this book. Their names are listed below. While their reflections were critical to our work, Pat and Suzanne alone take responsibility for the analysis presented here.

Wendy Winters has held the project together and has, as usual, made invaluable contributions at every stage of this project. Nancy Shannon transcribed with care more than five hundred interviews. Chermay Espino provided important assistance with the bibliography.

Those at McGill-Queen's University Press have been wonderful. Philip Cercone has been a strong supporter of our project. Ryan Van Huijstee produced a cover that delighted us. Kathleen Fraser sensitively edited the manuscript. Alexandra Peace produced the effective index. We thank them all.

Finally, we would like to thank our families and partners, who helped us in so many ways too long to list.

PARTICIPANTS IN ETHNOGRAPHIC RESEARCH
SITE VISITS, RE-IMAGINING LONG-TERM
RESIDENTIAL CARE MAJOR COLLABORATIVE
RESEARCH INITIATIVE

Adams, Annmarie	McGill University
Agotnes, Gudmund	Bergen University College
Armstrong, Hugh	Carleton University
Armstrong, Pat	York University
Baines, Donna	McMaster University
Banerjee, Albert	York University
Barken, Rachel	York University
Braedley, Susan	Carleton University
Chivers, Sally	Trent University
Choiniere, Jacqueline	York University
Daly, Tamara	York University
Davies, Megan	York University
Day, Suzanne	York University
Doupe, Malcolm	University of Manitoba
Erlandsson, Sara	Stockholm University
Goldmann, Monika	Technische Universität Dortmund
Heaslip, Ashley	University of British Columbia
Jacobsen, Frode	Bergen University College
James, Robert	York University
Kehoe MacLeod, Krystal	Carleton University
Kezirian, Alexis	University of British Columbia
Koneckis, Rilana	Technische Universität Dortmund
Kristiansen, Margrethe	The Arctic University of Norway
Lanoix, Monique	St Paul University
Lexchin, Joel	York University
Lloyd, Liz	University of Bristol
Lowndes, Ruth	York University
MacDonald, Martha	St Mary's University
McGregor, Margaret	University of British Columbia
McPherson, Kathryn	York University
Mekki, Tone Elin	Bergen University College
Meyn, Christina	Technische Universität Dortmund
Miles, Penny	University of Bristol
Müller, Beatrice	Philipp University of Marburg

Næss, Anders	Norwegian Social Research
Pallenberg, Vera	Technische Universität Dortmund
Panos, Justin	York University
Schulze Beiering, Marius	Technische Universität Dortmund
Smele, Sandra	York University
Sörensdotter, Renita	Stockholm University
Storm, Palle	Stockholm University
Stranz, Anneli	Stockholm University
Struthers, James	Trent University
Szebehely, Marta	Stockholm University
Theobald, Hildegard	University of Vechta
Vabö, Mia	Norwegian Social Research
Vaillancourt Rosenau, Pauline	University of Texas
Wenner, Judith	Technische Universität Dortmund

WASH, WEAR, AND CARE

Setting the Stage

Clothes are about class, culture, and care. And they are of course also about gender. More than an indicator of social position, clothes are critical to the "dignity of personal identity" (Bayer, Tadd, and Krajcik 2005, 22; see also Calnan, Badcott, and Woolhead 2006). Their condition reveals the care work that has gone into their selection and maintenance. But the maintenance especially remains largely invisible, in large measure because such care work has long been the responsibility of women as well as of some minority men, and is often hidden in the household (van Herk, 2002), in institutional basements, or behind closed shop doors.

This book is about that invisible laundry work and its relationship to the dignity of personal identity for both those who do the work and those who wear the clothes. Drawing on evidence from our current international study involving the UK, the US, Sweden, Norway, Germany, and Canada, we provide an analysis of both laundry labour and the importance of clothes in long-term residential care – a neglected social institution where even more neglected laundry work is done. Our objective is to explore what laundry and clothing can tell us about the experience of care and work in nursing homes, as well as about the wider social, political, economic, and historical contexts in which nursing homes are embedded. In the process, we raise larger theoretical and empirical questions about gender, racialization, work, care, policies, and the search for profit in neo-liberal times.

For our purposes, long-term residential care refers to facilities that provide around-the-clock nursing and personal support, are subject to some state regulation, and have some form of public funding. Most commonly called nursing homes, these facilities provide residents with more than what is usually understood as nursing care. They also offer assistance with activities of daily living such as eating, bathing, and dressing, access to physicians and other specialized health professionals, and social and recreation programs, as well as meals, housekeeping, and laundry services. The people who live in these homes have chronic conditions – ones that cannot be cured by modern medicine – and most have some form of dementia. As admission criteria have become increasingly restrictive, more and more nursing home residents require high levels of assistance with daily living as well as some medical care (OECD 2011). A growing number die within six months of entry. Although these facilities are still mainly places for older women, the closure of chronic care, rehabilitation, and psychiatric hospitals in many jurisdictions means that more residents now are male and more are younger. And across North America in particular, the resident population has also become more racially and culturally diverse. These places are called homes because people live there over the long term and because the emphasis is intended to be on the kind of care offered at home, often described as social care rather than as medical care. Not incidentally, calling them homes also allows governments to require residents to pay for their accommodation as they would at home.

Long-term residential care (LTRC) is where many of the most vulnerable live and, in spite of moves towards aging in place, where many will continue to live in the future. It is also a workplace for thousands of paid and unpaid providers, most of whom are women and many of whom are from racialized communities. It is a barometer of values and practices and a signal of economic, cultural, and social perspectives, raising issues that go beyond specific services and practices: issues such as human and social rights; the role of the state; responsibilities of individuals, families, and governments; work organization and skills; and notions of care. Nevertheless, in North America especially, nursing homes have received very little research attention and are low on the policy agenda.

The research that has been done on nursing homes has seldom examined clothes and their care, while the research done on laundry in health services has focused primarily on hospitals (Barrie 1994; Chau et al. 2010; Messing 1998b; Singh et al. 2009). Yet clothes have a particular significance in long-term residential care and so does their maintenance. Because these are homes, residents wear their own clothes. Just as in a home, clothes reflect residents' identities and their individuality as well as the ability to control how they are perceived by others (Twigg and Buse 2013). Clothes are particularly important as identifiers in this communal setting where so many processes are organized to promote conformity in ways that can undermine individuality. How residents are dressed can be the most significant indicator of their personality and of their life outside the nursing home. Clothes also indicate how much and what kinds of work have gone into their care.

Because these are care facilities, laundry is a part of the service and is subject to the processes within the facility. When residents enter, they are usually warned to bring only wash-and-wear, inexpensive clothes, and to label all clothing. This request may well mean a transformation in their clothing selection that challenges identity. Indeed, labelling itself marks a major transition from home to facility, one that can depress both residents and their families. Workers, too, are often required to wear certain kinds of clothing. Colour-coded uniforms that identify them with a particular place in the facility hierarchy are common, although some facilities allow workers to wear their own clothes based on the argument that this is a home.

Family members often take responsibility for the care of some clothing (Dempsey et al. 1993), especially if they would otherwise have to pay for part of the laundry service (Keefe and Fancey 2000) or if they are dissatisfied with how laundry is done at the facility (Ross, Carswell, and Dalziel 2001). Laundry can also be an important source of involvement for family members, who may perceive doing their relatives' laundry as a way to remain connected to their care (Habjanic and Pajkinhar 2013). Residents may also participate in laundry work, which can serve to involve them in a meaningful task and promote relationships between staff and residents (Taft et al. 1993). In order to encourage resident participation in the laundry process, laundry facilities can be modified to make them less confusing for persons with dementia (van Hoof et al., 2010). Volunteers may help with laundry as well, usually doing what family members would otherwise do.

However, the majority of dirty clothes are collected, transported, sorted, inspected, washed, dried, hung or folded, delivered, and stored by paid workers. Paid workers also usually play a major role in selecting the clothing to be worn by the resident each day, especially as more and more are very frail by the time they enter the nursing home. Increasingly, workers dress the resident, thus influencing not only which clothes are worn but also how clothes look when they are worn. Institutional rules and broader regulations cover these cleaning, selecting, and dressing processes. Most frequently, this means treating the clothes in the same way as soiled linens, and approaching both clothes and linens as they would be treated in hospitals.

Although often invisible, this laundry work has a critical influence on the dignity and health of residents. Dirty, wrinkled, lost, or shrunken clothing can undermine both health and self-respect, not to mention upset both the resident and their family. The laundry work process also has a profound impact on how the home looks and smells. Hallways crammed with carts of soiled linens look institutional and emit odours that permeate every room. Less visibly, laundry is an element of environmental cleaning, which plays a critical role in preventing infection outbreaks (Greig and Lee 2009). Equally important and equally ignored in the literature on residential care, the laundry work process structures the health and dignity of not only those who do the laundry but also those who do other kinds of work in the nursing home. Often concealed in a windowless basement and defined out of care, the health hazards too are often hidden away in remote laundry rooms, risking workers' health with needles, odours, and infection even when they have not had direct contact with residents (Standaert, Hutcheson, and Schaffner 1994).

Laundry involves complex and multistep processes for taking the dirty laundry away, for supplying clean laundry to the residence floor, and for ensuring it is in good condition – processes that require teamwork among all workers (Castle and Bost 2009). Laundry can support healthy, dignified personal care for nursing home residents when it runs smoothly (Goodwin 1994), but when it does not, it can also be a source of conflict in care relationships among workers, as well as with residents and family members (Austin et al. 2009; McGilton et al. 2008). Austin et al. (2009, 370) found that laundry is an "iconic" source of tension and conflict among residents, family members, and care staff. When family members are dissatisfied with laundry services (Ejaz et al. 2002; Moultrie et al. 2005), it is the frontline care workers who often have to answer to disappointed or angry family members (McGilton et al. 2008).

For several reasons, it is not easy to track what happens to laundry workers in nursing homes and to their work in the wake of neo-liberal reforms. One reason is the way statistical organizations compile data. Statistics Canada, for example, now reports workers by who employs them rather than by where they work. As a result, nursing home laundry workers now employed by a company that also services hotels would fall out of the health care category and into the personal service industry. Laundry workers are thus further defined out of care and even less visible in the data. Moreover, most of the data lumps together support workers to include laundry, dietary, and housekeeping in a single category. Another reason for the difficulty in sorting out laundry workers is the division of labour. Different jurisdictions and even different employers divide the work of laundry in different ways, and this division may change over time. Sometimes this work is done by care aides or even by nurses, sometimes by housekeeping, and sometimes by dietary aides, with the laundry added to their other tasks (Daly and Szebehely 2012).

WAYS OF SEEING CLOTHES AND LAUNDRY

This book is guided by feminist political economy, informed by theories of care. Like theory in general, this theoretical framework tells us where to look, how to look, and what to do with what we find.

Economics, politics, culture, and ideologies are understood within feminist political economy as integrally related, shaped by unequal forces of power and resistance differently in different historical periods and circumstances. Class, gender, race, and age – among other intersecting social relations of inequality – are critical to the analysis whether we are looking at international or local forces. This means asking which groups are affected in what ways, when, and under what conditions.

In the search for driving forces in current times, feminist political economy begins with how the pursuit of profit shapes social relations and institutions. This is not the only driving force but it is the most powerful. The extent of state support for the pursuit of profit varies both with history and with country, and all governments have put some limits on this pursuit, usually in response to demands from citizens' groups or workers' organizations. While the pursuit of profit and states' responses percolate throughout society, other forces also shape particular social relations and institutions. Feminist political economy means not only identifying the trends but also identifying the pressures behind these trends and asking whose interests are served by them. Context, structures, power, and resistance matter.

Feminist political economy assumes different, unequal, and conflicting interests. Indeed, conflicting interests are most frequently the basis for change. But change can itself create contradictory results, turning victories into losses or having opposing results. Moreover, what benefits some actors may not benefit others; what works for residents may not work for staff or for relatives of residents. Such tensions and contradictions are not restricted to those among groups, however. Some processes and relations may be contradictory in themselves – contradictions that need to be recognized and handled in the organization of care. A focus on tensions and contradictions moves us beyond dichotomies such as *good or bad* to ask how tensions can be balanced and how they lead to change.

Feminist political economy has focused particularly on women's work. It was feminists who insisted that notions of work include work that is unpaid, and who introduced the notion of social reproduction as central to understanding how systems develop and change (Armstrong and Armstrong 1978; Luxton 1980). From this perspective, the production of goods and services in the market is integrally related to the production of new paid workers on daily and generational bases as well as to the maintenance of the young, seniors, and disabled people who are not employed in the market. This daily work of feeding, clothing, dressing, caring, and having babies is women's work, work often hidden in the household or the community and absent from both theory and national accounts (Armstrong and Armstrong 1978; Luxton and Bezanson 2006; Vosko 2003). Gender, the dominance of the market, and the links between paid and unpaid work all contribute to the low value attached to women's work and to the skills that this work requires (Armstrong 2013). These forces can also contribute to the low value attached to seniors who are no longer working, most of whom are women. By emphasizing social reproduction, feminist political economy draws attention to the entire range of paid and unpaid work in the public and private sectors of the formal economy, in the community and in the household, as well as to divisions within these sectors (Armstrong and Armstrong 2005).

Not surprisingly given the emphasis on class in traditional political economy, feminist political economy began by exploring how class is gendered. However, it quickly became obvious that gender too is complicated by other relations of inequality and especially those of racialization (Connelly and Armstrong 1992; Bannerji 1995; Vosko 2003). As Dodson and Zincavage (2007, 921) point out, racialized workers are often seen by employers in this field as "uniquely suited to their jobs," coming from a "culture of respecting the elderly ... they are warm and patient ... they have that approach."

Such an analysis requires lumping and slicing: looking at what is experienced in common and what is not (Armstrong and Armstrong 2004). It means asking which women are the focus of any research and what are the differences among women as well as between women and men. In attending to these social relations, feminist political economy stresses the need to listen to those who do the work. The purpose is to understand what work women do, how they do that work, how they experience the work, and the consequences not only for them but also for their households. This approach is based on the assumption that workers have expertise, while recognizing that it is the researcher's job to locate that work and those understandings of work within broader social contexts (Smith 1987).

Feminist political economy also means taking collective and individual worker action into account along with the contradictions that often result. Workers' organizations have played an active role in providing some protections for paid workers in all the jurisdictions involved in our project, except for Texas where unions are uncommon. Even in Texas, however, those supporting workers' rights have managed to win some regulations such as minimum wages that provide limited forms of support. Although unions have helped to improve wages and working conditions for workers throughout the health care sector, government policies and regulations as well as union strategies have resulted in a wide variety of protections among jurisdictions.

This variation is particularly evident when it comes to defining scope of practices and competencies that stipulate who can do what (Daly and Szebehely 2012). In Ontario, for example, only licensed nurses can give most medications, and these nurses have fought hard to leave work such as laundry behind. Meanwhile in Sweden, those who do work similar to Canadian care aides can give many medications and combine personal support work with laundry and some cleaning. The result is contradictory. On the one hand, the Ontario-style regulations help protect both residents and workers by ensuring that the care providers have the necessary skills while limiting task shifting (Denton et al. 2014). On the other hand, the division of labour tends to separate medical and social care in ways that can harm residents, emphasize hierarchy in ways that can undermine teams, and leave some workers with a narrow range of repetitive tasks.

While feminist political economy draws attention to the gendered nature of work and the ways gender is complicated by other social relations, care theory focuses on understanding care as a relationship, albeit one that involves activities (Day 2013). This means understanding that "care is not an object. Nor is it a standardized or uniform product. It is, rather, a concept and an ideal that refers to both intangible affective/cognitive elements, and to observable, material actions which have clear consequences for each party involved" (Fine 2007, 143). Care work thus has a particular character that differentiates it from other forms of labour. It necessarily involves at least two people, both of whom are active in some form in what is often a reciprocal relationship. Unlike many other forms of labour, the timing and duration of care needs are often unpredictable and vary significantly over time of day and of life.

Taking a feminist political economy approach, Banerjee and Armstrong (2015, 11–12) identify four critical implications of understanding care as a relationship:

First, relationships are central to determining what good care means for any particular person ... Second, relationships are not only an outcome of good care they are a method of providing such care and doing so safely ... Third, as a relation, care is much more than the completion tasks. How tasks are performed also forms part of care as does what happens between these tasks.

Toileting, dressing, and feeding can be done in ways that enrich or alienate, dignify or humiliate both the one receiving and providing care ... Finally, the relationality of care extends beyond the resident and care worker dyad. Residents live in a nexus of relationships with sometimes competing interests that include not only their family members but also other residents, as well as inspectors, other careworkers, volunteers and administration. This renders care dynamic and unpredictable, not well suited to prescriptive rules, but rather requires empowering strategies that enable needs to be communicated and heard, as well as the autonomy to balance tensions as best as possible amidst intersecting relations.

Feminist political economists emphasize that care is a relationship characterized by power and inequality, shaped by both structures and resistance. It is also highly gendered, with the work of care both mainly allocated to women and assumed to come naturally to women. For women especially, caring about someone often means caring for them (Noddings 1984; Tronto 1993; Grant et al. 2004). What may well be a labour of love is still labour, however. In addition to supporting the many activities of daily living (Armstrong and Kitts 2004) and offering clinical care, this labour involves the work of fostering social relationships and providing both emotional and social support, as well as help navigating and managing care services (Rosenthal and Martin-Mathews 1999). Glenn (2010, 5) lumps these activities into three elements and argues that "All three types of caring labour are included to varying degrees in the job definitions of such occupations as nurses' aides, home care aides, and housekeeper or nannies. Each of these positions involves varying mixtures of the three elements of care, and, when done well, the work entails considerable (if unrecognized) physical, social and emotional skills." Doing the work well requires conditions that make relationships possible. As we make clear in our project, the conditions of work are the conditions of care.

This approach fits well with the literature on the determinants of health (Marmot and Wilkinson 2006). According to the Public Health Agency of Canada, these include income and social status, social support networks, education and literacy, employment/working conditions, social and physical environments, personal health practices and coping skills, biology and genetic endowment, gender, and culture, along with health services. Our approach differs from this literature in two ways. First, for us the determinants are not separate factors but rather are inextricably intertwined. Second, we see these determinants as also operating within health services, with implications for residents, workers, relatives, volunteers, and management. This means understanding clothes and laundry as critical factors in healthy, dignified care.

In sum, feminist political economy includes the entire range of work involved in care and understands care as a relationship. It locates that care within the context of global, regional, local, and institutional pressures, understanding those pressures as unequal in strength and consequences for those of different classes and genders as well as in other social locations. As Vosko (2003) points out, however, this theoretical approach is constantly developing with new research, and our own research is no exception. Like E.P. Thompson (1978, 43), we see research as a dialogue between theory and evidence.

WAYS OF PRODUCING EVIDENCE

The evidence for this book comes from our seven-year project entitled Re-imagining Long-Term Residential Care: An International Study of Promising Practices. Initially involving academics from the US, Canada, the UK, Germany, Sweden, and Norway along with union, community, and employer partners, the project has grown to include more than fifty students, post-doctoral fellows, and research associates. Funded for seven years by the Social Sciences and Humanities Research Council of Canada and with additional funding through the European Research Area in Aging project, we are searching for new ways of conceptualizing and organizing long-term residential care, learning from and with each other. Guided by feminist political economy, our objective is to identify promising practices that encourage dignity and respect for both providers and residents. For us, this means practices that understand care as a relationship with multiple players, practices that support differences and equity, and practices that promote active, healthy aging based on the recognition of different capacities. It also means paying attention to power and the search for profit, recognizing that context matters. We understand that promising practices may be singular practices found in only one location; they may also be ideas that have not yet been fully applied, or they may be broader approaches to care worth sharing, examining further and imitating, or ensuring they are avoided.

Our methods are complex, layered, and reflexive, allowing us to evolve in new ways. They are composed of three basic approaches to developing evidence: analytical mapping, literature reviews, and site-switching ethnography. We draw on all three aspects here and on the work of our entire team.

Our analytical mapping generates descriptions and analyses of what long-term residential care looks like in our many jurisdictions. This research provides us with the material to understand the importance of context and the forces at work structuring long-term residential care internationally, nationally, and locally. In Esping-Andersen's (1990) terms, our project included the social democratic states of Sweden and Norway, the corporatist state of Germany, and the liberal democratic states of Canada, the UK, and the United States. The different assumptions about the social right to care are evident in the public resources committed to long-term residential care, with Sweden and Norway devoting the largest share of their gross domestic product to care for the older population and the US the least (Baines and Armstrong 2015/16). While Germany devotes fewer public resources than either Canada or the UK, the compulsory insurance schemes ensure that nursing homes have significant funding. The overwhelming majority of nursing homes in the social democratic countries are either publicly owned or non-profit, in contrast to the significant and growing number of for-profit homes in the other countries involved in the project. The differences in both notions of social rights and the amount of funding were evident in staffing levels. Although exact comparisons are difficult to make, our research shows that staffing levels are highest in the social democratic countries (Harrington, Choiniere, et al. 2012), with Germany supplementing regular staffing with a large number of paid apprentices. One sign of the staffing differences is the large number of privately paid companions in North America, hired because family and friends saw there were not enough facility employees to provide care (Daly, Armstrong, and Lowndes 2015). The division of labour also varied, with the most flexible division in the social democratic countries (Daly and Szebehely 2012). In addition, differences were evident in the number and kind of regulations. According to our research, "countries with higher rates of privatization (mostly the liberal welfare regimes) have more standardized, complex and deterrence-based regulatory approaches" (Choiniere et al. 2016) and spend more on administration (Harrington et al. 2016). Differences were reflected in the design. All the residents had their own rooms in Norway, Sweden, and Germany, and in the case of Sweden many also had small kitchens in their rooms, while in North America and the UK, there were as many as four residents in a room.

There were also differences that did not map neatly onto the three categories of welfare states. With the exception of the United States, all the countries in our study have relatively high rates of unionization in this sector. In spite of this, wages tend to be low in the UK and Germany, with Canada and Norway paying relatively higher wages (Laxer et al. 2016). Part-time employment is common in all the countries involved in the project, but in Germany and the social democratic countries part-time employees have statutory benefits. There are also significant differences in the amount of training assistive personnel have now or are expected to have in the future and comparisons are difficult given the quite different education systems in the six countries. Germany and Norway in particular stress professionalization (Laxer et al. 2016).

At the same time, there are similarities across all the countries. In all of them, the labour force is primarily female, although more men are joining the long-term care workforce. Many of these men are from racialized and/or immigrant communities, as are a growing number of the female workers (Laxer 2015). And in all of the countries, the workers are getting older; so too is the resident population. In addition, all of the countries are facing pressures to move to more for-profit delivery and strategies. Our mapping documents what such privatization means, as we explore further in the next chapter.

The literature reviewed for the Re-imagining Long-Term Residential Care project covers four main themes: approaches to care, accountability, work organization, and financing as well as ownership. In addition, for this book we conducted a literature review of laundry work in general, and of laundry work more specifically both in all health services and in long-term residential care. This review demonstrated that laundry and clothing are neglected issues in long-term residential care, while also helping us to identify major themes for our analysis.

While the mapping and literature reviews are critical to our analysis in this book, here we draw primarily on evidence from our rapid site-switching ethnographies. This constantly developing strategy seeks to capture rich complexity rather than strictly comparative, single-factor data. We have completed studies of twenty-five long-term residential care homes, including at least two in each of the countries involved in the project.

Sites were selected for inclusion in the Re-imagining Long-Term Residential Care study based on key informant interviews, local knowledge, reasonable access, and facility approval. Key informants in all jurisdictions provided advice on what homes, based on what criteria, we should use as a way of studying promising practices. With this advice, we approached specific care homes for access. We researched their context and structure, conducted pre-interviews, and then took in a team of twelve researchers to observe and interview over a week, from 7:00 a.m. until midnight or later. Six different people spent four days in each of two units in the home, interviewing and observing the full range of actors involved in nursing home care: laundry, dietary, housekeeping, and nursing staff, physicians and therapists, managers and receptionists, residents, families, students on placement, volunteers, and privately hired companions. The interdisciplinary teams, some of whom have not worked in this area, brought fresh eyes to the study. Mid-visit the entire team met to discuss what we thought we had learned, what we needed to explore further, and what we were missing. We repeated this exercise again at the end of the visit. We developed an additional day-long visit at a second and sometimes a third site which we call a flash ethnography. Prepared with our background material and our information from the previously visited sites, we met with managers, and then fanned out to do interviews (both prearranged and serendipitous) and observations before meeting again with the managers to give feedback, ask questions, and clarify our interpretations. Each team included faculty and students from multiple countries, with a significant number from the local area to help us understand not only the language but also the culture; this brought fresh eyes to the research. The point was to share different perspectives while developing a detailed portrait from which we can all learn about promising practices. While we worked to provide consistency in our data gathering, we were also flexible in keeping with our search for promising practices.

The result is over five hundred interviews from the twenty-five sites, plus a host of field notes. With the site visit portion of the project complete, we are now sharing and analyzing the data together as a research team. Pat Armstrong participated in all but two of the site visits, and Suzanne Day participated in five of them across three countries. For the purposes of this book, we reviewed all the interview transcripts and every field note in search of any and all discussions of laundry and clothes. Many of our observations and interviews, and our theory, pointed to the critical contributions of laundry work to nursing home care. They graphically reveal how preventing loss and damage to residents' clothes, ensuring that residents have clean clothing and appropriate dress, and other laundry-related quality issues are all implicated in the provision of dignified, personalized care. And the way this work is organized, along with the conditions of work, has a profound impact on the dignity and health of those who do the laundry work, both paid and unpaid.

The project as a whole has ethics approval from York University, from other universities with faculty involved, and from the individual nursing homes, which have granted us access through their own internal approval processes. More details on our rapid, site-switching ethnography approach can be found in the appendices.

ANALYZING THE ETHNOGRAPHIC DATA

In the next chapter, we begin by bringing together our mapping and ethnographic data to analyze the context at multiple levels and to document who pays for and who profits from the way clothes and laundry are handled in long-term residential care. We explore how market strategies, justified as cost-saving measures amidst constrained health care resources (Government of New Brunswick 2013; Pullen 2015; Rashid 2013), influence the costs for paid workers and families, as well for governments. The adoption of privatization in various forms too often ignores both the critical role laundry plays in dignified care and the particular skills involved in nursing home laundry work (Armstrong et al. 2008; Cohen 2001; CUPE 2003). We saw a wide range of models for managing nursing home laundry across and within jurisdictions: some homes do all their own laundry, while others contract it all out; some contract out the linens but do the personal laundry in-house. The kind and location of equipment also varied, often in relation to the size of the residential units and the size of the facility as well as with ownership. We illustrate how it is not only the staff who pay in terms of lost security, lower compensation, and heavier workloads but also families and volunteers (Grant et al. 2004). We show how the costs of laundry are increasingly being downloaded onto residents and/or their relatives as a private expense, rendering laundry more marginal to the provision of care in nursing homes and widening class-based inequalities among residents. The example of laundry allows us to explore the implications for both workers and residents of encroaching privatization in health care services more generally.

This analysis sets the stage for our examination in chapter 2 of how laundry work is organized and of the division of labour that accompanies particular forms of organization. We also saw multiple, and often complex, ways of allocating and coordinating laundry tasks among those who did paid and unpaid laundry work and among people from different countries or racialized groups. While some homes have designated laundry workers, others assign laundry work to those who provide much of the personal care. Some encourage family care – especially from women in the family – while others make such contributions difficult. Family participation also varies with cultural backgrounds and class. The chapter ends with a discussion of the consequences these different forms of laundry organization have for both those who do the work and those who wear the clothes and sleep in the beds.

Chapter 3 looks at other kinds of costs created by the conditions of laundry work: namely, the risks to residents and workers. We explore how, in keeping with the medical model, laundry is approached primarily as an infection risk for residents (Barrie et al. 1994; Chau et al. 2010; CUPE 2003; Greig and Lee 2009). Although important in protecting the health of particularly vulnerable people, this approach reinforces the emphasis on the medical aspects of care. To the extent that laundry is understood as an infection issue, the treatment is the same as in hospitals and often ignores the unique features of residential care. As is the case in hospitals, the risks for workers of the laundry process and of work organization are not high on the agenda of research or policy. Yet, as we show in this chapter, our research reveals multiple and often severe health hazards faced every day by those who do laundry work – research that confirms and expands on evidence produced by others (Cohen 2001; Smith 2003; Thielen 2003). In addition to the physical risks are the mental ones resulting from repetitive, undervalued labour and the risk to relational care produced by the division of labour. We end the chapter by using our examination of laundry working conditions to raise broader questions about how risk and risk management shape care and work in nursing homes.

In chapter 4, we build on the evidence presented thus far to explore further how nursing home laundry and clothing can contribute to and undermine the identity, dignity, and well-being of both residents and workers. Drawing on additional evidence, we demonstrate how caring for clothing and laundry has important implications for the quality of care in nursing homes (Goodwin 1994) – particularly given the meaningful role that clothing can play in embodied memory and with the expression of identity for persons with cognitive impairments (Twigg and Buse 2013). We explore the relationship between laundry, clothing, and care from the perspectives of residents, their relatives, and nursing home workers, demonstrating how central laundry and clothing are to resident and worker well-being beyond the role that laundry plays in maintaining healthy environments. However, an overly narrow definition of care means laundry workers are often excluded from the wider care team and denied the rewards of relational care (Messing 1998b).

The failure to recognize the role of laundry and clothing in promoting respectful care and dignified work can result in an institutional approach that contradicts efforts to make these places resident-centred homes where people enjoy their work. In keeping with our theoretical framework, chapter 5 focuses on conflicts, contradictions, and tensions especially in relation to the emphasis on these places as homes devoted to resident-centred care. We explore the many ways the preferences of residents and families, along with the dignity of personal identity, can be undermined by regulations, working conditions, and laundry processes. For example, both workers and residents told us that the colour-coded uniforms we saw in many homes give an institutional feel to the place and emphasize hierarchy among staff. At the same time, uniforms can help both residents and families identify who is responsible for what and may provide dignity of identity to occupational groups. Doing laundry can create a feeling of being home, especially for women, who account for the majority of residents (Taft et al. 1993). But even when the appropriate equipment is available to allow residents to participate, a lack of staff, volunteer, or family time combined with regulations can prevent such participation and further undermine this idealized vision of home.

The concluding chapter draws out the lessons for laundry work in nursing homes and for thinking through approaches not only to care and care labour but also to conducting research. We argue that understanding nursing homes begins with those who live and work there, but also necessarily involves locating those experiences in the larger social, political, economic, and ideological contexts that shape them. In doing so, we seek to raise larger theoretical and methodological questions about care, about work, and about dignity for seniors.

1

Who Pays and Who Profits

Hardly a week goes by without a media story about the rising costs of health care, often accompanied by warnings that the grey tsunami will bankrupt the system. The solutions most frequently offered to this looming crisis resulting from a rapidly aging population are neo-liberal, with an accompanying emphasis on privatization and a market-based approach to health and long-term care. Although such strategies have been, and continue to be, promoted throughout the globe, they have been adopted to varying degrees and in different ways in different jurisdictions. In Norway, for example, nursing homes have long been understood as integral to the universal welfare system, and they remain primarily public, based on a counter-ideology of public provision and backed by a strong economy (Jacobsen and Mekki 2012). Yet in Norway too there are pressures to adopt privatization strategies and some moves have been taken in this direction (Vabo et al. 2013). When clothes and laundry are defined out of care they are particularly vulnerable to privatization, even when they are understood as part of the service in nursing homes. In this chapter, we begin by looking in more detail at neo-liberal approaches before moving on to explore how these approaches are applied to clothes and laundry. We end by illustrating the costs to workers, residents, families, and nursing homes in terms of expenditures, time, and care.

NEO-LIBERAL APPROACHES

In the 1970s, global developments started to reshape long-term residential care in North America and the UK. The oil crisis, stagflation, government debts, and labour unrest contributed to a move away from the post–World War II consensus based on Keynesian economics that supported economic regulation and a strong welfare state. Theorists like Hayek (1944) and Friedman (1962) promoted small government, free markets, and competition as the way forward, an approach that Thatcher in the UK, Reagan in the US, and to a lesser extent Mulroney in Canada enthusiastically embraced. Within governments, there was a move towards New Public Management. In an approach that can be summed up as "private is better than public" (Kapucu 2006, 887), New Public Management promoted reducing government by outsourcing or abandoning services, by applying competition and market strategies to the services that remain or that government funds, and by entering public-private partnerships. The specific applications varied from country to country but even the Nordic countries joined the parade (Kamp and Hvid 2012; Meagher and Szebehely 2013), as did Germany (Van de Walle and Hammerschmid 2011), each following somewhat different paths. All governments in the countries included in our project used both policy and expenditure tools to support marketization in some forms. Yet all of them have simultaneously supported and constrained the application of neo-liberal approaches, and have done so in different ways.

From a neo-liberal perspective, the innovation and efficiency needed to meet the growing demand for seniors' care could best be achieved through market competition and private-sector managerial strategies (Prada 2011). Competition would improve quality and efficiency and thus save money while also expanding choice. The market was assumed to provide most of the necessary regulation, but there was also an emphasis within the public sector on performance management, outcomes measurement, and what has been labelled an audit culture (Power 1999). Focusing on workers and to some extent their employers, accountability was understood narrowly as counting and reporting on counting.

These neo-liberal notions became increasingly popular just as governments were increasingly concerned about rising health care costs. This concern coincided with falling profits in old industries and searches by corporations for new sites of investment. For example, the business and investment company Forbes (Tice 2014) promoted home health care on its website as "a hot niche, with relatively low investment and high revenue." At the same time, there was growing opposi-

tion to what was characterized as institutionalization and medicaliza-
tion, to the overreliance on placing people in large facilities, and to
over-treating within facilities (Sheth 2009). Technologies too were
changing, making it possible to transfer significant aspects of care
from inpatient to outpatient services and to provide more treatments
outside of hospitals.

APPLYING NEO-LIBERAL SOLUTIONS TO HEALTH CARE

In response to this combination of pressures, and to varying degrees
among jurisdictions, governments have applied market strategies to
health services. They have justified such strategies in terms of popular
support for both change and choice, claiming as well as that this
approach was required to save the public system. Hospitals were amal-
gamated based on the assumption that large firms are more efficient.
Chronic care, rehabilitation, and psychiatric hospitals were closed,
based on the argument that their patients would be better served in
the community. More surgeries were done on an outpatient basis and
more complicated medical care was sent home, most often to be provided by women without formal training or pay. Managerial
approaches taken from the for-profit sector were increasingly applied
to the public-sector organizations that remained (Armstrong and Armstrong 2016; Kamp and Hvid 2012; Meagher and Szebehely 2013).
Even in mainly public systems, more costs were transferred to individuals, based largely on the argument that this would promote more
responsible use of health services.

Such strategies to define public health services more narrowly and
to reorganize them had a direct impact on the population entering
nursing homes. More of the residents had significant mental health
issues, more had chronic diseases requiring complex medical care,
more were incontinent, more had mobility issues, more were men,
and more were younger, at least in North America. This major shift in
population made the work heavier, harder, and more challenging for
everyone, including for those looking after clothes and laundry.

The freeing of international markets alongside state cutbacks has
also encouraged the global movement of workers across borders, especially from low-income to high-income countries (Eckenwiler 2012).
Many of these global workers are women who have few options in

their home countries and very limited options in the countries involved in our project. Because they are women, it is assumed they can do women's work, and much of health care has long been defined as women's work. Because much of the work, and especially the work of cooking, cleaning, doing laundry, and providing direct care – such as help with eating, bathing, dressing, and toileting – involves labour traditionally defined as women's work, many migrant care workers find employment in nursing homes. Because they are not in their countries of birth, their credentials from home are not often recognized in the employing country, so they take this work even though they often have training for other jobs (Kofman and Raghuram 2006).

Unions have provided some protections against the impact of neo-liberal developments. Among the sites involved in our project, all workers, except those in the US, were represented by unions. Nurses have been more successful than others in protecting their skills and, at times, their jobs. These providers have fought hard to shed parts of the job such as dressing, changing diapers, and doing laundry, allowing them to focus on what they see as the skilled components of the job (Armstrong and Armstrong 2009). But with the application of New Public Management, they too have seen many of their jobs disappear and their work become intensified while more have found only part-time and/or casual work. The emphasis on debts and deficits, rising health care expenditures, and labour costs as the primary component in public health care funding have all worked against union gains. Indeed, unions themselves have been under attack, in part blamed for driving up costs through workers' gains. It is a combination that is hard for unions to fight successfully, especially in the face of governments using public opinion and temporary workers as a means to undermine collective strength. Unions have been more successful in Germany and in Nordic countries, where strong unions and strong economies have helped protect workers from some but not all of these developments.

APPLYING NEO-LIBERAL SOLUTIONS TO NURSING HOMES

According to the Organization for Economic Cooperation and Development (OECD 2011, 1), "There is a history in many countries of [long-term care] policies being developed in a piecemeal manner, responding to immediate political or financial problems, rather than being constructed in a sustainable, transparent manner." Until relatively recently, nursing homes have been a mix of charitable and government-owned facilities along with some generally small, privately owned ones that reflected such piecemeal development. The Nordic countries did develop universal public elder care services beginning in the 1950s but they were "developed on the basis of housewifely skills and virtues; those who worked in the sector were typically housewives, who based their work on their identity and experience as housewives" (Kamp and Hvid 2012, 13).

In North America especially, such facilities mainly served the frail elderly, most of whom were women and many of whom were poor. Those with medical needs were cared for primarily in hospitals, some of which specialized in psychiatric, rehabilitation, or chronic care services. Those who needed long-term care were on the periphery, the neglected edge of the health care system. Nursing homes were often seen as places of failure: the failure of individuals to care for themselves, the failure of families to provide care for them, and the failure of the health system to cure them. It was better not to think about them and avoid them at all costs, which people could do if they had enough money to pay for private, twenty-four-hour care. Serving such a population based on such assumptions and with care provided mainly by women, long-term residential care has been a low-wage and low-status sector.

By contrast, in the Nordic countries "different and better conditions have been established for developing meaningful work, whose contribution to society is recognized on a par with other professional work" (Kamp and Hvid 2012, 13). Yet in these countries too governments have embraced New Public Management strategies. In their book on elderly care in these countries, Kamp and Hvid (2012, 14) demonstrate how this "sector has become a testing ground for neo-liberal management."

In this context, neo-liberal strategies reflect and shape approaches to care in nursing homes. They also have a profound influence on who owns nursing homes, who provides the services within them, and how these services are provided. We turn now to explore these strategies and their impact on laundry and clothes as well as on those who do the laundry and wear the clothes.

THE IMPACT ON APPROACHES TO CARE

Medical models focus on biological factors as well as on diagnosis, treatment, and the doctor as expert, supported by trained, licensed, and regulated nurses. This model has fit well with many neo-liberal approaches, as well as with an elaborate, hierarchical division of labour. Increasingly, medicine has "given primacy to targets, narrow and specialized outcome, technology, efficiency drives, and audit pathways" (Galvin and Todres 2013, 1). Although in nursing homes the emphasis is intended to be on the non-medical aspects encompassed by the term social care, such as assistance with daily living and emotional support, medical care often takes priority and the medical approach can shape how the work is organized. Getting the clinical aspects right becomes a priority, and those in charge are primarily trained in clinical work. Such an approach fits well with efforts to define laundry, dietary, and housekeeping services as hotel services that are particularly amenable to for-profit managerial strategies. This notion was made explicit in a Commission on the Future of Health Care in Canada, which argued that "a line should be drawn between ancillary and direct health care services and that direct health care services should be delivered in public and not-for-profit health care facilities" (Romanow 2002, 7).

Yet defining such services out of care contradicts the social determinants of health literature that understands health as structured in and outside a nursing home by a range of factors that include laundry, housekeeping, and dietary work (Wilkinson and Marmot 1998; Armstrong, Armstrong, and Scott-Dixon 2008). Indeed, these services are even more important to the health of particularly vulnerable populations such as those in residential care. Soiled sheets and clothes, as well as badly prepared food and dirty environments, are not only dangerous to the physical health of those already in weakened conditions; they are also harmful to dignity and self-worth. The contrast between management and family understandings of the role clothes and laundry play was particularly evident in one Canadian province. When we met with senior management and a couple of governing board members at one long-term care home, we raised the question of laundry towards the end of our two-hour meeting. A female board member who had not yet spoken immediately jumped in to tell a story of her mother's sweater, lost for months and returned destroyed. A female social worker talked about how laundry had been raised as an issue regularly in resident council meetings. We had heard such complaints many times before, but what was particularly interesting to hear was the director's response. He intervened to quickly cut off the discussion that ensued, telling us firmly to move on to more important issues. Urging participants to "not make a mountain out of a molehill," he suggested that problems with laundry and clothing were marginal to the other aspects of care in the home. The combination of neo-liberal approaches, the medical model, and the growing demand for residential care contributes to a focus in laundry research on saving money through market means and on preventing infection. The cost of laundry is characterized as a major problem and reducing laundry cost has become a common objective. As acuity levels among residents increase, so too do the demands placed on a facility's laundry services (Castle and Bost 2009). Incontinence is seen as a major cause of this growing demand (Borrie and Davidson 1992; Cummings et al. 1995; Hu, Kaltreider, and Iguo 1990) – one that is more often understood as a medical issue than as a social one.

As we explore more fully in later chapters, how governments and homes respond to this increasing demand has a profound effect on both residents and workers. While cutting laundry costs by switching to disposable diapers (Cummings et al. 1995; Hu, Kaltreider, and Iguo 1990), for example, may in the short term save some spending on chemicals, water, and staff time, this comes at the incalculable expense of undermining the comfort and dignity of residents. In contrast, investing in staff to implement continence programs (Borrie and Davidson 1992) can not only save money on laundry in the long term, but also enhance the dignity of residents and make relational care more possible. Especially in North America, privatization strategies are evident in various forms, as we discuss in the next section.

PRIVATE OWNERSHIP

One response to the cost pressure and to demands for neo-liberal strategies is to hand the entire nursing home to for-profit owners. Indeed, some jurisdictions have actively encouraged the for-profit ownership of nursing homes.

A health minister in British Columbia was explicit about his government's support for the involvement of the for-profit sector in nursing homes: "It's historically been a partnership and that partnership needs to continue, and looking forward, I see real opportunities for the private sector" (Goodsell 2012). The private sector invited to partner with government is almost always corporate, consisting of large, investor-owned chains that drive out small, often family-owned operations. The Ontario government was less explicit at the same time as it developed what is best described as an affirmative action plan for corporate ownership (Armstrong, Armstrong, and Kehoe MacLeod 2015). In the late 1990s, the government announced a competitive bidding process to build 20,000 new LTRC home beds and retrofit another 16,000 to meet safety, fire, and privacy standards (McKay 2003a; 2003b). The request for proposals did not explicitly favour for-profit corporate chains, but the competition process did so. Those bidding were required to have access to enough capital to build new buildings or massively refit old ones. Small, family-owned companies did not have the capital to invest in such projects and neither did most charitable organizations or cash-strapped municipalities. The elaborate proposals required not only considerable preparation time but also expertise in preparing bids. Small municipal and charitable homes, as well as small privately owned ones, did not meet these necessary conditions, either because they had no infrastructure or because they did not have the experience to deal with the competitive process. Moreover, new standards relating to the physical structure were hard for those owning older buildings to meet out of current revenue. As a result, two-thirds of the 20,000 new nursing home beds were awarded to for-profit nursing home chains. The top five municipal and charity-based nursing home operators were awarded 2,049 new beds while the top five for-profit companies were allocated 6,573 new beds (McKay 2003a). As of 2015 (Ontario Auditor General 2015, figure 1), 53 per cent of the beds are in for-profit hands.

Corporate ownership of nursing homes is less common in Scandinavian countries than it is in North America and the UK, but Scandinavian countries are not immune. In Sweden in 2012, "21% of the beds in residential care [were] provided by the private sector" (Erlandson et al. 2013, 27). The competitive tendering, with quality rather than price the major criterion, "favoured larger companies, since they have a greater capacity to handle the paperwork related to tendering than small companies or non-profit organizations, and they can also underbid, if necessary, to enter the market" (Erlandson et al. 2013, 48). In Norway, "competitive tendering was introduced in the late 1990s" (Vabo et al. 2013, 181), with the nature of the process varying by region. However, Norway has not gone nearly as far as other countries in privatizing ownership. Vabo and colleagues (2013, 195) argue that this reflects a number of factors: "the need for cost reduction has been lower," given the way oil and gas revenues have been invested; "marketization is mainly an instrument suited to densely populated areas" and Norway has a small population; and "Norway's strong consensus culture and well-organized power of resistance are important reasons for the relatively moderate level of marketization."

It is not surprising that corporations are anxious to enter the field of nursing home care. The demand is growing and, at least in the countries in our study, governments basically guarantee payment and even subsidize construction as well as guaranteeing virtually full occupancy. It is more surprising that governments keep supporting the move to corporate ownership, given the evidence that they do not provide cheaper, better care or more choice. According to a Canadian study, "compared with for-profit chain facilities in Ontario, non-profit, charitable and public facilities had a one-and-a-half to two times lower chance of receiving a verified complaint" (McGregor et al. 2011, e188). A verified complaint is one that has been followed up by the ministry to ensure it is reasonable. The highest number of such complaints were made against for-profit chains, accounting for 47.4 per cent of all complaints (McGregor et al. 2011, table 3). The majority of the verified complaints were about resident care (McGregor et al. 2011, table 2). Such a large number of complaints is particularly worrisome given that the auditor general (2015, 369) reports that inspectors "often did not take timely action to ensure residents were safe and their rights were protected" after complaints were received. "In another jurisdiction (Fraser Health, BC) non-profit facilities had a three to four times lower chance of receiving a complaint compared to for-profit facilities for total and substantiated complaints respectively" (McGregor et al. 2011, e188). Complaints in BC must be substantiated by the community licensing office in order to be counted. A third of the complaints were about care and staff and half the facilities accounted for all of the substantiated complaints. As was the case in Ontario, chains and larger facilities accounted for relatively more complaints.

Differences in verified complaints are not the only indicators of poorer quality in for-profit homes. An Ontario study examined mortality rates and transfers to hospitals in publicly funded long-term residential care facilities (Tanuseputro et al. 2015). This research found significantly higher rates of mortality and of hospital admission in for-profit homes compared to non-profit ones.

Research in Canada (Hsu et al. 2016; McGregor et al. 2011), the US (Harrington 2013), and Sweden (Stolt, Blonquist, and Winblas 2011) also indicates that for-profit chains have the lowest staffing levels. And staffing levels are directly and indirectly linked to the quality of care (Castle 2008; Schnelle et al. 2004). That McGregor and colleagues (2005) found slightly lower laundry staffing levels in non-profit compared to for-profit facilities may reflect the attempt in non-profit homes to provide more integrated care through a more limited division of labour. Increases in nursing staff levels have been found to be associated with declining levels of support staff, including laundry workers (Bowblis and Hyer 2013), suggesting a possible "substitution" effect as laundry shifts onto nursing staff. It is thus not surprising that when offered a choice among homes, Ontario residents clearly prefer to avoid for-profit nursing homes. Ministry data from 2010 indicate that 67 per cent of first choices were for non-profit and municipal homes, although they together account for only 46 per cent of the homes and the fees are the same as in for-profit homes (Buchanan 2011).

At the same time as governments have been facilitating corporate ownership or public-private partnerships and supporting free markets, they have also been pushed to place limits on how these owners operate. Unions, citizens' organizations, and the media have all played a role in demanding such limits – limits made even more necessary by privatization. A study of nursing home scandals in all of the countries involved in our project found that "for-profit residential care provision as well as international trends in the ownership and financing of nursing homes were factors in the emergence of all media scandals, as was investigative reporting and a lack of consensus around the role of the state in the delivery of residential care" (Lloyd et al. 2014, 2). The main response to scandals has been more and more detailed regulations and more documentation, ostensibly in the name of public accountability. Not surprisingly given the differences in ownership patterns, detailed regulations and documentation requirements are much more likely in North America where corporate ownership is common. Such detailed regulations, however, have focused mainly on workers and workplaces, leaving larger structural questions such as ownership and staffing levels largely untouched (Banerjee and Armstrong 2015). As a result, the consequences of union pressure and scandal exposure have often been to put more restrictions on workers and to create more work for them in documenting the minute and daily details of care. These trends are in keeping with New Public Management notions of accountability.

Chains have been active in opposing regulations that can influence their bottom line, however. Forbes (Tice 2014) puts it quite succinctly on its website: "National chains also have the money to do lobbying and advocate for favorable laws – most recently, against the proposed federal minimum wage increase." Although the article is about corporations in the US, their success in lobbying shapes all nursing homes in many countries because competition requires a race to the bottom.

Moreover, governments do little about corporate decisions to move or close facilities. And some go bankrupt. Yet again, Ontario offers a number of examples. In 1997, Lakeview Nursing Home, located in the small upper Ottawa Valley town of Cobden, was closed by the for-profit owner and the licence transferred to construct a facility in another, larger town hundreds of kilometres away. The town meeting, required by legislation, objected strongly to the closure because it would mean residents could no longer be housed in their community and fifty people would be put out of work, but the transfer happened anyway. The minister responsible said there was little the government can do if an owner wants to close. Indeed, ministry officials approved all requested transfers out of the home that was closing, but access to care and family near the home was gone (Egan 1997a; 1997b). Southern Cross offers a UK example. With the government's approval, the corporation expanded to own hundreds of nursing homes, but this search for profit ended with bankruptcy. One of those homes was accused of "institutionalised abuse" by the coroner investigating the deaths of five residents (Milmo 2013), even though it had a good rating from the government inspection team. The intensified turmoil resulting from the Southern Cross bankruptcy and takeovers meant increased anxiety about care quality for its 37,000 residents and increased anxiety about job security for the workers caring for them (Scourfield 2011).

Based on her many years of studying the consequences of nursing home ownership in the United States, Charlene Harrington (2013, 237) concludes that "profit margins are obtained by controlling staffing levels and labor market costs at the expense of quality." And, we could add, at the expense of workers. For-profit LTRC facilities are more likely than their non-profit counterparts to have poorer wages, fewer if any benefits, and weaker collective agreements (Canadian Healthcare Association 2009).

CONTRACTING OUT

Privatization has not stopped with the ownership of nursing homes, however. Most commonly in North America, governments have also supported or even required the contracting out of services within charitable, non-profit, or government homes that receive public funding. Laundry, housekeeping, dietary, security, and even management services have been outsourced (Daly 2015). In spite of research demonstrating the critical and specific roles these services play in health care (Armstrong, Armstrong, and Scott-Dixon 2008), they have been defined out of care in order to justify contracting them out to corporations that serve hotels or other industries. As is the case with new ownership, such contracts usually go to large, international corporations such as Sodexho, often meaning the relocation of services outside the facility.

Such contracting out frequently means work that is more precarious in terms of job security, pay, benefits, and other protections, as research in BC demonstrates (Zuberi and Ptashnick 2011). In their systematic review of the impact of contracting out on workers, Vrangbaek and colleagues (2015) report that the negative consequences dominate. They point out that the lack of security also often means experienced workers are replaced by younger workers.

The application of an industrial model to such health services assumes that separating out tasks such as laundry reduces the skill requirement and thus the rewards necessary for the work (Braverman

1974). Training can suffer as a result, with consequences for infection control and workplace injuries (Zuberi and Ptashnick 2011). This is especially the case when the work is separated physically and socially from that of other workers, as it usually is with the privatization of services. Most of these workers are women and many are from racialized and/or immigrant communities, workers who often have limited power (Laxer 2015).

The promises of cheaper, better services and more choice from such contracting out are seldom realized. According to a Saskatchewan study (Grant, Pandey, and Townsend 2014, 4),

> Three reasons are given why the promised savings and efficiency gains from privatization or out-sourcing may not be achieved: (a) quality shading, where privatization results in a lower quality of service; (b) redistribution, where privatization yields no efficiency gains but merely redistributes income from workers to the government and the private firm's shareholders; and (c) hold-up costs, where the private firm deliberately understates the initial costs and then seeks to ratchet up the price of the contract to the government once public production facilities have been closed.

It is also argued that governments do not have the money to invest in new laundry or other services. As Interior Health's regional director of support services in BC put it, "It's about avoiding future significant spending to replace aging equipment, an investment we can't make when considering other health-care medical equipment priorities" (quoted in Hynd 2015). Yet relying on private money necessarily costs more money in the long run, mortgaging the future to avoid current expenditures on the public accounts but without the advantage of owning the equipment in the end (Whiteside, 2015).

As the UK Public Services International Research Unit (2014, 4) puts it, the "results are remarkably consistent across all sectors and all forms of privatisation and outsourcing: there is no empirical evidence that the private sector is intrinsically more efficient." Indeed, the "Hospital Employees Union in B.C. found that payments to two laundry corporations that hold the monopoly on service to health authorities in the Lower Mainland increased by a staggering 170 per cent over a seven-year period" (Donaldson and Stadnichuk, 2015).

Privatization does not mean more efficiency but it does mean less transparency. Although public dollars pay for what the public services corporations deliver, these corporations claim that their finances must remain secret in order to remain competitive. Governments and health authorities regularly support such claims. When the Canadian Union of Public Employees sought a copy of a Saskatchewan linen contract, the union received a copy of the ten-year contract with many essential components blacked out. The good news is that the Saskatchewan Information and Privacy Commissioner (2015) recommended that the full contract be provided. The bad news is that such contracts still remain secret in many jurisdictions. Even though governments often claim commitment to transparency and stress auditing systems, the secrecy involved in private ownership and contracting out contradicts these claims and prevents the public assessment of both quality and working conditions. Marketization also means democratic power is diminished. As Meagher and Szebehely (2013, 283) put it in the case of Nordic countries, the introduction of publicly funded, for-profit ownership "established new interest groups in welfare politics, with potential to influence the direction of policy."

In sum, rapidly running out of new places to invest, those seeking profit have recognized that the aging population throughout most of the world offers an opportunity for new markets, and have worked hard to ensure that conditions allow private investment in these new markets (Prada 2011). Fears fanned by population aging and by mounting public debts and deficits provide fertile ground for the privatization push that includes the adoption of for-profit managerial strategies within public services. As Meagher and Szebehely (2013, 273) explain in their discussion of marketization of Nordic eldercare, many of the preconditions necessary for markets to work do not exist in health services and there has been remarkably little research on the impact of market approaches on care. "Health care is not a business like the rest and those working in health care differ in some significant ways from those employed in other sectors" (Armstrong and Armstrong 2004, 118). It is about life, death, and individuals, which means that risks cannot be primarily assessed in economic terms. Health care is also an interactive process among individuals, one that necessarily requires that context be taken into account and that relationships continually change. Partly in response to pressure from unions and from popular groups and to failures in neo-liberal strategies, governments have simultaneously supported and constrained the application of neo-liberal approaches to care. There are significant variations among countries in the extent to which they have applied marketization approaches. Nevertheless, all have adopted some of these practices and introduced new forms of accountability based on counting. And all of this has a variety of negative consequences for families, for residents, and for workers.

COSTS FOR RESIDENTS AND FAMILIES

While in later chapters we explore in more detail how families and residents are involved in clothes and laundry, here we want to highlight how this involvement has changed with new austerity measures and with the application of neo-liberal strategies to care. Their changing involvement is viewed as another form of privatization, a shifting of responsibility from employers and governments to individuals. Especially in North America and the UK, residents and families have long taken some responsibility for their clothes and laundry. They have helped pay for and maintain personal clothing, although they seldom take responsibility for linens or other materials used by the facility. With privatization, however, costs in time and care have risen.

Health systems and health system funding vary significantly across and even within jurisdictions in our study, but in all of them, governments provide funding for residential care, and in all of them residents are required to pay some of the costs. The justification for these payments is also similar across jurisdictions. As Stephen Duckett (2012, 132), a former health services manager in Canada and Australia, explains: "part of the service there directly substitutes for a home (that would otherwise be paid for by the resident as rent or capital) and for the food, light, and power that would normally be paid for by the individual. But some services – health care provided by nurses and other staff such as personal care workers – are not a substitute." It is a fuzzy distinction. In our publicly funded hospitals, these "direct substitutes for a home" are defined as part of the care in the Canada Health Act (Government of Canada 1984), with laundry as well as food, light, and power all considered integral to the service. The distinction seems to hinge on the definition of these facilities as homes or residences where people live for long periods of time, as opposed to the short-term, acute care services of a hospital. It also seems to relate to a distinction between medical and social care, with the emphasis theoretically on social care in nursing homes. It is a distinction that is increasingly difficult to maintain as stricter admission criteria mean more of those in nursing homes require complex medical care, more live in these homes for shorter and shorter periods of time, and more have numerous and severe physical and cognitive impairments. Purchasing personal clothes can be defined out of care, but keeping them free of infection and treating them when people are incontinent can be defined as medical. Moreover, as we see in more detail in the next chapter, the complex division of laundry work in most nursing homes makes it difficult to sort out the costs of collecting, sorting, transporting, washing, drying, and returning clothes from other services that "are not a substitute."

However, it is clear that more care is being defined as a substitute and that neo-liberal approaches can create more work for families as a consequence. For example, low staffing levels that accompany privatization, especially when combined with rigid regulations, can mean residents spend most of their time in wheelchairs. According to a Vancouver family member we interviewed, his mother walked into the home upon admission but was immediately put in a wheelchair because there was not enough staff to ensure safe walking. As a result his mother now needs different clothes, ones that work in a wheelchair, cost more than her previous wardrobe, and bear little relation to the clothes she once picked out for herself. Staffing also influences toileting, and toileting has an impact on clothes. As an RN explained, "getting help to the bathroom at the time that I want – that is another big issue." The failure to respond to requests to get to the toilet means more soiled, smellier, and more damaged clothes. It thus means not only more laundry but also either different clothes that can withstand chemicals and resist stains or undignified clothes, as we explore in greater detail in chapter 4.

In addition, the application of corporate strategies to food can shape what clothes can be worn and are required. In a Nova Scotia for-profit home, a daughter complained that the industrial kitchen in another municipality produced such starch-laden food that her mother gained weight all the time and thus constantly required new clothes. When this daughter sought different food, she was told the only option was a diabetic diet which was even more boring and was rejected by her mother.

Most of the female family members of residents we talked to in North America did the personal laundry for their relatives, especially if they had access to laundry facilities at home. But Canadian research suggests that families are more likely to take the laundry home if they would otherwise have to pay for some laundry services, indicating class plays a role (Keefe and Fancey 2000). In a Texas for-profit home, management explained that "we just charge you a monthly fee based on your incontinence level ... Some of them bring their own and bring them into the community" as a way of reducing their fees. But we learned there were similar fees in the non-profit home we visited, as the care aide explained: "If you need a diaper or toothpaste, they can give it to you but you get something else. You know what it is? It is a bill! They write it down quick. So people provide sheets, towels, diaper or Depends, toothpaste, snacks. If they provide, they charge you." She went on to say that this means each resident's clothes and linens are washed separately because "You can't have the pissy sheets of you touch the pissy sheets of Mr over there. No, no!" (said with humour).

With various privatization strategies, however, families may have little choice but to take on the costs of laundry themselves. The adoption of industrial laundry processes of the sort we saw most commonly in North America often wrecks clothes, either forcing families to buy new ones or encouraging them to take the laundry home. Low staffing levels mean there is less time to take care in handling clothes. Lack of staff has encouraged many families in the homes we visited to hire private companions to ensure their relatives were properly dressed and their clothes handled with care. We saw wide variations in the presence of such private companions, providing one indicator of gaps in care. They were most common in Canadian homes serving residents from higher income groups. However, we did see some in the Nordic countries and were told their numbers were growing as marketization strategies took hold. One Ontario home put washing machines and dryers on each floor for private use and made it clear that some clothing would not be the responsibility of the nursing home. This strategy did at least mean women did not have to lug the laundry home and back, and it did allow those without laundry facilities at home to do the work for their relatives – if they had the time and were physically able. Residents without family or the financial means to hire someone to do the work simply had to give up any clothing that would not withstand the industrial process.

It is not only families but also volunteers who are called on to take up the slack that results from austerity and privatization. Once more this was primarily the case in North America, where volunteers substituted for family members in taking on the extra laundry work and the work of providing clothes.

In sum, neo-liberal strategies have cost consequences for families. Especially in North America, it is not new for families to ensure their relatives have clothes and that these clothes are maintained. However, a variety of changes in staffing and other ways of organizing work have given families less choice in doing this work and more work to do. It is mainly women family members who take up the slack. At the same time, lower staffing levels also have an impact on how residents are dressed and on the extent to which their personal dignity as reflected in their clothing is maintained. The impact is greatest on those who do not have relatives with the time, money, or physical ability to provide the additional care work. These residents are most likely to be female not only because they are the majority but also because they are the majority without economic resources to compensate for the consequences of privatization.

COSTS FOR WORKERS

Workers, too, often pay for the application of neo-liberal strategies to clothes and to laundry labour, as we show in greater detail in the next chapters. They pay in terms of job security, benefits, and wages as well as in terms of job satisfaction and health. They are not alone, however. The regional economy may also suffer as a result.

Privatization in the form of either corporate ownership or contracting out produces the most obvious costs for laundry workers. Most of the nursing homes we visited had centralized laundry for towels, napkins, and linens and many of those centralized laundries were operated by corporations. When laundry is outsourced it can mean that the job leaves as well. We heard from more than one worker in Canada that the union was not able to protect them from con-

tracting out. Even if the workers employed by the contracting company had a union, contracting itself often undermined the union's
power to protect workers or their skills. The contracted workers
belonged to a different union than that of the workers in the contracting home, and belonging to a different union with a different
employer limits the possibility of working in teams and of feeling like
a member of the team.

Such privatization often leads not only to lower wages, reduced
benefits, and job insecurity but also to a narrower range of repetitive
tasks and exclusion from the wider care team (Armstrong, Armstrong,
and Scott-Dixon 2008; Cohen 2001; Stinson, Pollak, and Cohen 2005).
A BC study starkly illustrates what happens when such laundry and
cleaning services are outsourced: "In less than 10 months – from October 2003 to July 2004 – all housekeeping services in the 32 hospital
and extended care facilities in southwestern BC were contracted out to
three of the largest multi-national service corporations in the world –
Compass, Sodexho, and Aramark. The impact on wages and working
conditions was immediate and stunning: wages for the privatized
housekeepers were cut almost in half, benefits were eliminated or
drastically reduced, and union protections abolished" (Cohen 2006,
626). Pay equity gains were also eliminated, restoring the gender-
specific wage discrimination that had been previously demonstrated
and addressed.

A Saskatchewan study of health services laundry privatization in
Prince Albert estimated the costs as "74 jobs lost in the region, a
decline in labour income of $2.5 million in the region, and a decline
in regional GDP of $3.7 million" (Grant, Pandey, and Townsend 2014,
20). These estimates do not include all the ripple effects on local shops
and services, nor do they include the cost to the environment of ship-
ping laundry long distances on a regular basis.

Some workers retain their union status when there are new owners. But unions may have difficulty maintaining old protections
when services are privatized. As a US study of health care laundry privatization showed, unions became less powerful even when they
retained their members in the newly privatized workplace (Ness and
Zullo 2003). The study found that "when workers are unionized, collective bargaining transfers to a less favorable legal and political context, shifting the balance of power toward management." Concession

bargaining that resulted in lower wages also resulted in more divisions among workers.

Even when laundry work remains in-house, the threat of privatization and the pressure to reduce costs has an impact. In one Ontario home, the laundry staff was told that an evening shift was to be added as a way of preventing privatization through cost savings on water. Two workers would be assigned to that shift. A laundry worker's initial reaction was positive: "I thought 'Oh, wonderful. Wonderful. We'll have time to actually get the job finished to the way we were taught, to the way we expect it to be.' And it's just like oh no, they're going to put the laundry in the evening shift as well and then you're going to have bed making and then you're going to have stuff that wasn't originally your job but is now your job." Not only was the job expanded but the number of workers was reduced to one who laboured alone. Moreover, the evening shift disrupted her home life: "For the evening shift I had to re-arrange all appointments. I was not there for dinner. I was not there for evening entertainment like movies or what not. I wasn't there for that. That was the biggest complaint. I wasn't there for that. It was only six months but six months too soon when we really didn't ... it seemed like you're making progress, but then part of the progress they make it doesn't seem like they're making progress in some areas. It's just the way they re-arrange things and they re-arrange our lives." A Vancouver home faced similar pressures as the government cut back its funding. The director explained that she currently has only one main laundry worker in her medium-sized nursing home. As a result, "the workload is very heavy because every single day we're not just washing towels, facecloths, blah, blah, blah, or linens. We have to do a lot of personals because nothing is contracted. Everything is in-house." The director there was also contemplating reorganizing the work to integrate laundry into other care work in order to cut costs. She made it clear that this would be possible to do because she saw the work as requiring few skills. However, she did not know if this would happen because the union was resisting this move.

In a Canadian for-profit nursing home on the east coast, the worker pays for the consequences of privatization in the form of unpaid overtime. There, the dirty laundry is taken from the rooms in large carts and sorted into different containers in the soiled linen closet. The clients' clothes go in with all the other laundry and come out wrinkled. Because a woman we interviewed is "from the old school," describing the clothes as "my clothes" and explaining, "I wouldn't want to see my mother" in wrinkled clothes, she irons residents' laundry on her own time.

There are benefits to doing laundry in-house, benefits to both the people who do laundry and those who wear the clothes. A director of a non-profit Canadian home provided a description of laundry work and workers that identifies these benefits.

DIRECTOR: Yeah, so that's sort of a good thing. Because [name] is always the person doing it and she's always involved on the floor the residents are really comfortable with her. One of the deals is everyone in the building has to know the residents and so everybody's job incorporates at some point in that day they have to spend some time doing something with the residents.

INTERVIEWER: So you don't contract out anything other than the washing of the bed linens?

DIRECTOR: No. We do everything in-house. We cook our own food. We have our own housekeeping staff. The only contracts that we have [are] the physician and the pharmacist.

A laundry worker in that home compared working for both a private and a public nursing home and told us she felt more respected in the public facility.

WORKER: The other one was private. The other one you had … management I've got to say was probably on the same lines but nurses were a little bit different. Here I guess maybe because it's government that they really treat you differently I guess with more respect. They don't consider themselves way above.

INTERVIEWER: The nurses or the management?

WORKER: Both. The management at the private and the management here were almost about the same but here it's probably a little bit more open and stuff like that. But then you're going from 215 to 80 [residents], right, so there's a lot less staff and you would see a lot less people during the day so you'd have more time to communicate, right? But yeah, I would say the nurses are a big issue with that one. But here they're different.

For this worker, public ownership leads not only to fewer residents but also to better relationships among staff.

In sum, various forms of privatization and cutbacks in the public sector cost workers in terms of pay, job security, benefits, social relations, and, as we shall see in the following chapters, health. And they can cost the local economy as well.

CONCLUSIONS

Laundry work has never been highly paid, highly valued, very healthy, or recognized as skilled. Especially in North America, women in families have taken some responsibility for providing clothes and for maintaining them in long-term care. With various forms of privatization, however, those costs to workers and families have increased. Even in Sweden where the state has assumed more of the responsibility in the past, there is a growing expectation that families will pay for clothes being cleaned and that workers will add laundry to their regular workloads without new training or a lessening of other tasks. This chapter sets out some of the economic and political forces shaping long-term care and describes some of the costs. Subsequent chapters expand on these costs as they play out in the daily lives of residents, families, and workers.

2

The Labour of Laundry and Clothing

Clothes take a lot of work, especially if those wearing the clothes are frail and have dementia along with limited mobility. Clothes have to be purchased and selected to be worn each day, to fit not only the person and their preferences but also their activities during different times of the day and seasons. In most long-term care homes they have to be labelled with the resident's name and room number. Clothes also have to be put on and, given that most residents require partial or total help getting in and out of their clothes, the work of dressing takes on a particular form in residential care. In addition, clothes have to accommodate the care work, regulations, and other requirements associated with this form of communal living. This clothing work takes time, resources, and many hands. And this is in addition to the more obvious fact that clothes have to be stored and kept clean, processes that require sorting, transporting, washing, drying, ironing, and folding as well as returning them to their proper place.

But clothes do not account for all the laundry. Bed linens, towels, and other materials produce dirty, stained, soiled, and smelly laundry that also needs to be transported, sorted, washed, dried, folded, and returned. In other words, as van Herk notes, "laundry must be 'done'" (2002, 894) – meaning, of course, that someone has to do it. This daily labour of laundry is essential to maintaining the appearance, cleanliness, and comfort of residents' clothing and, by extension, of the residents. Nursing home brochures typically inform residents and their family members that the laundry is included in nursing home services. However, there are often suggestions that families may want to take care of more delicate items, and there are usually instructions about what kinds of clothes to bring in order to accommodate the home's laundry services.

It takes many different kinds of work and the work of many different people to ensure that nursing home residents are dressed appropriately and with dignity, and that the beds are clean for residents to sleep in throughout the day and night. Examining the clothes and laundry labour in nursing homes entails not only the question of how the work is organized and who does it, but also what the underlying conceptual frameworks are that inform this work organization. Indeed, looking at the labour involved in laundry and clothing can tell us a great deal about the work of nursing homes more broadly.

Building on the analysis in the previous chapter, we explore here the different forms of work organization and labour processes related to laundry and clothing within a context of neo-liberalism, the medical model of care, and the application of market-based logic. These are not the only influences, however. Gender, racialization, historical practices, union struggles, ideas about skill, and government regulations, as well as local managerial practices, all shape the organization and processes of labour. Families also play a critical role. Indeed, the unpaid work of families both complicates the work organization and differentiates work organization in nursing homes from other workplaces. Not surprisingly, given these pressures, we saw no single predominant model for organizing laundry and clothing work in nursing homes. Nevertheless, we can identify two broad approaches to work organization that emerge from this context – approaches that have been identified as characteristic of neo-liberalism. One is the detailed, hierarchical division of labour characteristic of an earlier period but reconfigured in various ways with privatization. Such an approach enhances the power and skill of those at the top while often dismissing the skill and limiting the autonomy of those at the bottom. As Braverman (1974) observed, the application of this industrial model to work organization often results in the deskilling and degradation of labour. Under the assumption that dividing up the labour reduces the skills associated with the work as well as the time required to learn the job, it thus justifies lower rewards as well as a speed-up of the work. Equally important, such a strategy can increase an employer's control over the work and the worker. Under this approach, clothing and laundry work are assigned to different workers, with laundry understood as among the least skilled tasks followed closely by other work with clothes. Applying this model can also undermine teamwork and integrated care focused on the resident. However, as Braverman's critics such as Beechey (1982) made clear, the model focused on deskilling fails to take reskilling, worker resistance, non-industrial workplaces, and gender into account. As is the case in many workplaces, there can be positive consequences of the detailed division of labour. For example, in health care this division can help ensure that those assigned clinical work have the required skills and that responsibilities are clear. It can also allow some workers relative autonomy as they go about their work (Witz 1990), making the work more satisfying for both those providing and those needing care.

A second approach to work organization is the flexible division of labour, based to a large extent on the notion of the generic worker (Rolfe et al. 1999; Sky 1995). As MacDonald (1991, 179) explained, this approach "held out a promise of more holistic jobs, a reversal of the increasingly detailed division of labour – in short, the promise of more satisfying, rewarding work for more people." It seems particularly promising in health care. With this approach, care labour is organized to incorporate the work of laundry and clothing, combining it with other labour. This can mean more integrated care, more teamwork, and a more homelike atmosphere. However, under market-based logic focused on efficiency and cost savings, the result is often expanded workloads, a failure to recognize workers' skills, and negative consequences for the well-being of both workers and residents. In short, these different approaches have different and often contradictory consequences, as we suggest in the following sections. It should be noted, however, that these approaches do not appear in pure form and are more complicated in practice. Moreover, with the exception of those we call registered nurses, the classification of workers varies across jurisdictions and so do their qualifications (Harrington, Choiniere, et al. 2012; Laxer et al. 2016). Nevertheless, using these two categories allows us to see both the broad frames that organize work and the pressures that shape labour in the specific case of nursing homes.

At the same time as we saw significant differences in work organization across and within jurisdictions, we also saw some common patterns related to gender and racialization. In all of the jurisdictions in our study, nine out of ten people paid to do care work are women, and women also do the majority of daily unpaid health care (Laxer 2013). To a large extent, this reflects a shared assumption that it is work most women can do by virtue of being women, part of the inherent "nature" of women (Leira and Saraceno 2002). This is particularly the case for assistive personnel. Although "some sub-units have more extensive professional requirements for assistive personnel" (Laxer et al. 2016, 65), suggesting a growing recognition of skills that need to be learned, all jurisdictions have a history of hiring women without much reference to formal qualifications of the sort that are often used to define skills, and generally the certification and education levels of assistive personnel are low (Laxer et al. 2016). The limited application of consistent formal requirements makes it harder to define this work as skilled and to protect the conditions that allow workers to use their skills (Armstrong 2013). It does, however, make it easier to hire those women from immigrant and/or racialized communities who have difficulty getting their formal credentials recognized, based on the assumption that any woman can do the work.

THE HIERARCHIES OF CARE: NARROWING THE JOB AND THE VALUE OF THE JOB

More commonly in the North American sites we visited, laundry and clothing work is organized according to a complex and hierarchical division of labour. This division of labour is gendered, racialized, and classed. Within this context, the organization and valuing of work is most often based on the assumption that clothing and laundry are ancillary to clinical care.

Placing the labour of laundry and clothes near the bottom of the hierarchy and defining it as unskilled fits with a medical model that separates clinical and social care. But the division of labour also reflects workers' struggles to gain recognition for their skills and to ensure that workers have the skills they need for the job. It is a division of labour also shaped by privatization and by regulations, as well as by managerial practices within the public sector. It is a division that is clearest with laundry and that becomes less clear as we consider clothing more broadly.

Registered nurses (RNs) and those variously called registered practical nurses (RPNs) or licensed practical nurses (LPNs), among other terms used in North America, have worked hard to carve out a space that ensures their skills are learned and recognized, no simple task for a female-dominated occupation long understood as a labour of love (Armstrong and Silas 2014). Often called regulated health professionals because their work is sanctioned by both governments and their own governing bodies, their strict admission criteria help account for the limited number of immigrants in this job category (Das Gupta, Hagey, and Turritin 2007). Nevertheless, the number from racialized and immigrant groups has been growing along with demand, and these numbers are greater in nursing homes than in hospitals, reflecting the higher pay in hospitals and the higher demand in nursing homes (Laxer 2015).

Nurses have also struggled to eliminate from their job descriptions work such as clothing and laundry, seeing it as ancillary to care and long defined as unskilled women's work (Armstrong et al. 2008). Usually as a result of nurses' collective efforts, in many North American jurisdictions, nurses in long-term care are the only ones who can give particular medications and do other clinical procedures. Nursing home regulations in most jurisdictions also require that a nurse be on duty and that a nurse submit the documentation that is part of the growing auditing system. RNs are usually the ones in charge not only of the unit but also of the home. Typically, RN responsibilities are listed as including connecting with the doctor; conducting complex clinical assessments; doing Quality Assurance related to wound care, infection control, falls, palliative procedures, etc.; referrals; and directing other staff. In other words, their focus is increasingly clinical and managerial.*

Also known as nurses, LPNs' job descriptions in North America involve them directly in auditing functions related to care plans, performing nursing care, directing assistive personnel, and administering medications and treatments. Unlike RNs, however, their job descrip-

---

*These and other job descriptions are taken from specific collective agreements. Although collective agreements are public documents, identifying a particular agreement would identify the nursing home, something that our ethics protocol forbids.

tions also refer to personal care. Personal care is broadly defined and encompasses the majority of the work done for residents in nursing homes. Regardless of job descriptions, we saw only a few nurses or other health professionals helping with clothes or laundry. This division fits with a medical model of care, as LPNs and RPNs occupy increasingly medicalized and auditing roles in nursing home care while RNs provide clinical and managerial oversight (Armstrong et al. 2009).

Under this model, the paid work involving clothes falls mainly to those frontline workers variously termed personal support workers, nursing aides, personal care assistants, assistant nurses, etc. These workers, whom the World Health Organization (2010) calls care assistants, are often unlicensed and closely supervised (Day 2014). The job description from one Canadian home reflects those of many: "Directs and assist[s] residents with all aspects of personal hygiene, including bathing, washing, bowel and bladder care, dressing, caring for teeth, hair, nails, skin, etc. according to individual resident ADL [activities of daily living] Care plans." There are at least two features to note in this brief description. One is that assistive personnel are only allowed to direct the residents, those who are often the least powerful in the nursing home, and not to direct other workers. Another is that the work of clothes is reduced to dressing in this description. Yet in practice these workers select the clothing to wear, making decisions about what clothing will look best on a resident and be most appropriate and most convenient at a specific time. They help residents to put on and take off clothing or do it for them if the resident is physically impaired or immobile, and they decide when clothing should be changed. Some of these workers also ensure that residents have sufficient clothing.

The clothing work of assistive personnel is shaped not only by the clothes available and by the preferences of residents but also by regulations about when and how people are dressed, by the time available to do the work, and by pressure from relatives as well as from the nurses who are in charge. Time poverty, created by heavier workloads resulting from increased complexity in residents' care needs, inadequate staffing, increased reporting requirements, and the division of labour, limits workers' ability to use their skills in dressing residents. This was the most common complaint we heard from both workers and families. Asked about taking care with dressing and grooming, a female worker in Ontario reported that "we can't do that. We don't have the time. They're like a number. Next, next, next." A limited wardrobe can also make the work difficult, especially if residents frequently soil their clothing and if workers do not have enough time to take residents to the toilet. The requirement at one home that residents be dressed and at breakfast by 8:30 a.m. means there is little time for clothes selection or dignified dressing strategies, especially when one of these workers has five residents to dress, as an Ontario worker explained: "Then we start work here because we have to get them up for breakfast ... You have to make sure that they're dressed. We take them out here [at] 8:30 ... You have to get them up in time. What we do, we don't have time to dress all of them who [are] having a bath so I'll put on your dusters or the shirts before they go and they have breakfast. Then we give them a shower or a bath after." Families, we were told, regularly complain about the way their relatives are dressed, adding to the pressure. At the same time, a detailed division of labour that puts nurses in charge and that severely limits what assistive personnel can do independently reinforces the notion that the work involves limited skills, as this Texas worker explains:

> Everybody [is watching you]. They do. I don't know, but somebody will report you somewhere. But we're used to it. You know, we're used to it ... If I get written up I get like three days without pay if you really, really did something bad. Whatever you do, you know, and they judge you on that ... We don't work the way we want. You know, everybody is watching us 24/7. We report everything to a nurse. Anything even small. So it's not like we are at home and we can do whatever we want. At the end of the day whatever we do is what we sign in. If we go above that we're going to get big trouble. Even go to jail for that. So everybody knows why they're here.

Like nurses, the overwhelming majority of assistive personnel in nursing homes are women. As is the case with much of women's domestic work, their clothing labour is often invisible and is mainly noticed when it is not done or is done badly. It is frequently treated as secondary to the "real" labour of clinical care and viewed as labour that requires little skill (Armstrong et al. 2009). More training and registration have been promoted as a way to enhance the skills of these workers and as a way of addressing the increasingly complex health needs of the residents. However, especially in North America we were told workers were expected to do most of the training that resulted in formal qualifications on their own time. Few of these women, with low wages and work demands at home, had the time or resources to do so. Training provided by the employer tended to be through the internet, something the workers we interviewed saw as of little practical value. Workers also worried that the skills they had developed through long years of practice would be devalued if registration was required.

Formal credentials fail to capture the kind of informal learning that happens daily on the job. We saw workers teaching each other how to handle individual residents and informing each other about dress preferences. They shared their knowledge about which resident likes their socks on first and who was most likely to get upset when colours do not match. They planned when they needed to work together to dress a difficult resident. At the same time, many of them have taken multiple relevant courses that are not recognized in their current jobs.

Many assistive personnel have joined unions as a way of improving their pay, benefits, safety, and job security. However, these unions have not tended to focus on protecting skills, as the nurses have. Although they have taken up issues of workloads, they have not often been successful in these efforts. It has proven difficult to resist cost-cutting strategies that focus on clinical care and attach much less value to the less visible social care that includes clothes. In addition, the low value attached to nursing home care in North America, where all of the residents are outside the labour force forever, where the overwhelming majority of residents are women, and where many of the residents have little income, contributes to the limited power of these workers.

The division of labour is more complicated when it comes to laundry, even in nursing homes characterized by a detailed division of labour. Privatized laundry tends to be an extreme form of the detailed division of labour. In the nursing homes we studied it was common to contract out the laundry for towels and linens, where the work was done under factory-like conditions by those exclusively involved in laundry work. This still leaves the clothes laundry to be done on site, although some homes even transport this laundry work to be done elsewhere. Designated on-site laundry workers at the homes we visited were either employees of the home or employees of the contracted company. For instance, we visited nursing homes in Texas and Manitoba with their own laundries, and the laundry workers were employees of the home. Both these medium-sized homes of nearly two hundred residents had only one laundry worker for the entire facility. A larger home in BC that had privatized laundry also had designated laundry workers on site, with at least two women on each shift.

Although the job descriptions of laundry workers often simply said "do laundry work," one Canadian job description captured much more of the labour involved:

- Sorts, folds, distributes, weighs and records linen and resident clothing.
- Issues linen and maintains records. Loads and unloads commercial washers and dryers, operates same for selected wash cycles and switches machines on and off.
- Checks and requests restocking of laundry supplies from designated supervisor.
- Does minor repairs to linens and to resident clothing.
- Sends residents clothing to dry cleaning.
- Labels resident personal and facility laundry.
- Irons resident clothes and linens.
- Cleans the laundry room and equipment, monitors equipment operation and reports any problems to designated supervisor.

It should be noted that very few of the homes we visited considered repairing clothes, ironing, or sending laundry for dry cleaning part of their responsibility, even though these are essential components in laundry work.

There are few if any formal credentials required for laundry jobs, although regulations related to laundry processes make it clear that knowledge is required to do the work well and safely. Indeed, specialized laundry workers do receive on-the-job training about safety and, like the assistive personnel, teach each other as they go about their work, as we will see in the next chapter.

Like assistive personnel, it is common for designated in-house laundry workers to belong to a union as a way of protecting their pay, benefits, and workloads. In Norway and Sweden, most contract details are centrally negotiated, which contributes to union strength. But in Canada each union negotiates with each employer, which can limit their power. Most laundry workers belong to the same union as assistive personnel if they have the same employer, but contracting out can mean different employers, and thus different contracts. With so much pressure to cut costs, unions have found it difficult to protect their jobs and skills.

Specialized laundry workers could mean that clothes are appropriately laundered by people with recognized skills, and work could be organized to ensure these employees are part of the care team. Indeed, we did visit a nursing home in Manitoba where the laundry worker took pride in her work and gained considerable satisfaction from developing relationships with residents as she picked up and delivered their clothes. The manager in this home was committed to involving all employees with residents on a daily basis and, because she was the first manager in this home, was able to hire employees based on this approach. A detailed division of labour that includes designated laundry workers can also offer pathways into employment and training. For example, in a UK nursing home we were told that laundry work offered a way to start in long-term care for those who had little formal education. A worker we interviewed explained that she received training for a wide range of laundry issues. The training either happened during her paid work time or was paid for if she came in for training on her days off. Once she had trained for this job and had worked in it for a while, she had the opportunity to move into other occupational categories. Moreover, specialized laundry work can serve as an entry point for immigrants whose credentials for other jobs are not recognized. As we heard, when laundry workers are direct employees of the nursing home, the job can provide a starting point on the ladder of the detailed vision of labour.

Under a detailed division of labour, there are boundaries. Laundry workers, for example, do not take off residents' dirty clothes, and often they do perform other work around the nursing home. As a UK worker put it: "Some places it's like laundry is laundry. Housekeeping is housekeeping. No mix. All very, very separate." This kind of strict division of labour focuses workers on a narrow range of tasks and was most common in the North American homes we visited. In addition, there is a high degree of variation in the boundaries specialized laundry workers face, depending on the kinds of other staff that the facility employs, the size of the facility, the kinds of equipment available to do the laundry, and the underlying models of care upon which the facility operates. For example, laundry facilities on each floor make it easier to assign laundry to assistive personnel while the location of laundry facilities in the basement makes it more likely there will be designated, and isolated, laundry workers.

But even when there are specialized laundry workers and a formal division of labour, we also saw a wide variety of additional in-house staff participating in the complex and multi-step process for making sure that there is clean clothing and linen for all residents in the facility. Laundry work requires teamwork among various types of workers and among and across different departments in the nursing home (Castle and Bost 2009). Assistive personnel especially are usually involved in at least some aspects of laundry work. For instance, at sites in Ontario and Manitoba, we observed frontline care workers collect and bundle soiled laundry and linens. In Texas, much of the laundry was done on the floor by the assistive personnel. In various Canadian sites, cleaners also participate in laundry along with other work crucial to maintaining the appearance and sanitation of health care settings (Messing 1998b). In some places they are responsible for the entire laundry process in the absence of designated laundry workers. In other words, laundry work is not only performed by persons who hold the job title of "laundry worker," even in places with the most detailed division of labour. Regardless of whether laundry is performed in-house or outsourced, a range of other workers are involved in the choreography of ensuring residents' clothes, dining room linens, and beds are clean.

Sharing the work of clothes and laundry can promote teams. However, the shared nature of laundry and clothing work does not in general extend to nursing staff. In our interviews in North America, we were repeatedly told that LPNs had, in the past, often helped with such work but new auditing systems were reinforcing hierarchy and taking nurses away from the personal care included in their job descriptions. The result was less rather than more teamwork unless, as we saw in one Canadian and one UK site, the director had an explicit policy requiring everyone to pitch in to get the work done.

In sum, in the detailed division of labour approach, the work of clothing and laundry is assigned to those lowest in the hierarchy, to those with the least formal credentials, and to those assumed to have the least skill. It is often treated as a starting point on the pathway to the relatively better-paying positions in the nursing home. Too often, the work of laundry and clothing is seen as a type of "dirty work" (Twigg 2000; 2002), and in its association with dirt, domestic servitude, and unskilled women's work, laundry has historically been accorded very low occupational prestige (van Herk 2002). Done primarily by assistive personnel, laundry workers, and cleaners, this work tends to be poorly paid and primarily performed by women – many of whom are from racialized and/or immigrant communities as care labour is increasingly sourced from the Global South (Eckenwiler 2012). Indeed, the proportion of immigrant and/or racialized communities increases towards the bottom of the hierarchy. Unionization in Canada has helped improve conditions, but the Texas workers we interviewed had no such support.

Looking at who does the work of clothing and laundry in places with a detailed division of labour reveals the gendered, classed, and racialized division of labour in nursing homes. It also reveals the underlying diverse and complex work organization even in these homes, demonstrating that such work must be done regardless of whether it is assumed that clinical care is the main job and that a detailed division of labour is efficient. Although the detailed division of labour does ensure some skills are protected and recognized, it leaves others with little power and few recognized skills while dividing up care in ways that can deny a focus on residents as people for whom dress and clean sheets are critical to both comfort and dignity.

A FLEXIBLE DIVISION OF LABOUR: EXPANDING THE WORK

A second approach to work organization in neo-liberalism is the expansion of workers' roles. Removing rigid divisions of labour is a central feature of the culture-change movement, which advocates expanding the job of assistive personnel to officially incorporate cleaning and laundry, tasks usually defined as domestic or housekeeping services. The main idea is to create generic workers who can perform a variety of tasks, ostensibly in support of a homelike atmosphere by eliminating strictly defined, institution-like divisions of labour and allowing for more integrated, person-centred care (Bowers et al. 2009). Flexibility can also mean less hierarchy and the promotion of teams. However, as noted by Daly and Szebehely (2012), within a neo-liberal context of constrained resources for care, the trend of expanding workers' job definitions may in practice be experienced as a downloading of additional work, causing significant problems for workers who are already struggling to manage unsustainable workloads. Furthermore, as Hallgrimsdottir et al. (2008) make clear, the downloading of care work tends to occur along gendered pathways, and thus disproportionately affects those workers who perform women's traditional domestic work in long-term residential care. Laundry and clothes work exemplify one area where this downloading occurs, with often negative consequences of this trend for both workers and residents.

Historically, flexible work organization has been more common in Scandinavian and German nursing homes than in North America, as has been more involvement of nurses in direct care. Based on a comparative survey of Nordic and Canadian workers, Daly and Sezebehely (2012, 143) reported that the Swedish care workers (both ANs [like LPNs] and CAs [assistive personnel]) carried out a variety of tasks, including not only cleaning, cooking, and laundry, but also recreation and other "social activities," which in the Canadian context were, to a large extent, carried out by other occupational groups such as dietary and activation workers and professional therapists.

In the Nordic countries, we saw many examples of teamwork that involved the entire range of nursing home workers, and team meetings that included those who do laundry and cleaning in addition to those who do the nursing care. We also saw workers with considerable autonomy in doing the clothing and laundry tasks as well as more integrated, relational care. In a Norwegian home, care workers take residents shopping for clothes and the time involved in doing so can be accumulated to provide paid time off. In a Swedish home, a worker would help a resident get up, get dressed, and take her medications. She would fill the washing machine in the room and would chat and clean the room while the wash was being done. But workloads have been even further expanded in some homes we visited, often undermining some of the advantages associated with a more flexible division of labour.

In line with a market model approach to care, expanding workers' jobs to include additional laundry work appears to be influenced as much by a cost-saving imperative as by a concern for creating a home-like atmosphere. For instance, at one Ontario facility, frontline care workers spoke to us about having their jobs expanded to include the task of sorting clean laundry and returning it to residents, eliminating the job of nursing home porters and thereby reducing the labour costs of the home. These care workers are now expected to find a way to fit this additional task into their already overwhelmingly busy shifts, which becomes a source of frustration and conflict when the job cannot be accomplished in one shift and has to be passed onto the next. At a Norwegian facility, the job of washing all of the residents' laundry as well as of cleaning residents' rooms was downloaded onto assistive personnel when the facility shifted from public to private ownership. This shift has had negative consequences for both workers and residents, as a care worker explained to us when she was asked about her tasks and how they had changed: "Now if you are disciplined and if you work correctly and hard every day, maybe it's okay. But I should have [a] little more time for the residents, because now we clean. Before we had a cleaner. But now everything we must do. And sometimes we say of course this is not so important that it's clean. It's better that we take care of the residents, but the family come and sometimes the floor is so dirty, and so you clean it." It is not only cleaning that has been added to her job but also the auditing work: "And we must document. Every day, three or four times every week, and this takes time with the computer. All of us are not so used to using the computer so it take a long time." Asked when the cleaner was taken away, she said, "I think when we privatized. And even the clothes. We have three [unheard] and three trousers, and you must clean them yourself, and you must change every day, and you must clean." The result is "much cleaning" that involves "towels, their clothes, residents' clothes, everything. Before we wash only the residents' clothes, but the towels and the bedding we put in the box ... So everything now we must do it."

When laundry services were eliminated, along with the cleaning staff, the duties of assistive personnel at this nursing home expanded significantly – as did their workloads. These workers now must wash all towels, bedding, and personal clothes of the residents, as well as clean the room; as a result, they have less time to spend with residents, and increasingly find their time is focused on workload completion. As others (e.g. Armstrong et al. 2009) have noted, social care is one of the first things that care workers will drop in response to workload constraints, often resulting in care that increasingly resembles an assembly line, becoming a task-oriented process as workers must prioritize certain tasks above others amidst unmanageable work assignments.

It is not that taking on laundry and clothing work constitutes an inherent problem in the reorganization of care work towards a more flexible division of labour. Indeed, it could mean more integrated care, more teamwork, and more job variety as well as greater autonomy for both worker and resident. Rather, what makes a difference is whether changes to the scope of direct care work are accompanied by sufficient supports and resources to manage the additional workload, and whether the skills involved in the work are recognized. For instance, assistive personnel at one Norwegian nursing home identified some positive aspects of taking on a portion of the laundry work, as this presented them with a way of dealing with the problem of lost laundry. At this nursing home, responsibility for laundering personal clothing has over time been shifted onto direct care workers, using in-unit laundry rooms. Speaking through a translator, these workers explained how the shift in the division of labour helped them to deal with the time-consuming problem of missing clothing:

> So it works quite well actually. Of course there is [unheard] but at the same time they have a system for dark clothes. Also when they put the washer on the floor it was beneficial in that they actually know where the clothes are now, because sometimes if you send it to the [centralized] laundry they disappear, and so the relatives, they come and ask, and also you have to work to find out where the lost clothes went. So now they have control. They know where the clothes are. They're in the washing room. So it's not so bad. Yeah, they have quite a good system to know where to put each resident's clothes so they don't have to go looking for it. They just can go to the spot where it's supposed to be.

Care workers at this nursing home seem to appreciate how this shift provides a means of control over the problem of lost clothing, saving them both the problem of conflict with family members and the work of hunting down missing items, as well as allowing them to pay more attention to how specific items are washed. In this sense, taking on laundry work has indeed helped care workers to support a "person-centred" model of care (Bowers et al. 2009). In Germany, an assistive care worker explained how this flexibility worked for her: "Every day is different ... If I need assistance I get it ... We have a lot of freedom (possibilities) ... If I wanted to work night shifts, I could do that. In this facility we work very cooperative; if I approach my boss about something if I want to change something, he will listen. And if it is at all possible, my wishes will be fulfilled." However, Norwegian workers also told us that laundry increased the burden of their workload as staffing levels were not simultaneously increased when this new task was added. Promises from the management that personal laundry would be outsourced have yet to materialize. Hence shuffling responsibility for laundry work is not itself an inherent problem, but rather it is the lack of support, resources, and training necessary for workers to handle the addition of new tasks.

Beyond the issue of workloads, the above experiences also raise questions about the skills required for care. It requires a significant amount of skill, knowledge, and training to do laundry in health care settings properly (Armstrong, Armstrong, and Scott-Dixon 2008; Cohen 2001; Stinson, Pollak, and Cohen 2005). Referring to a Swedish home, field notes summarize this issue that arises in the blurred division of labour: "The staff here do all the work required in the home, including cleaning the lift and dispensing the medicines to residents. A broad spectrum of skills is required. It does support the idea of the home as a household, which could add to the sense of home, but could it also mean that the staff come to resemble an all-purpose service, with less recognition of their skills?"

If the blurring means a denigration of skills and an increase in multitasking and staff workloads, then it is a problem for workers and residents. If it means expanding the range of skills and tasks and it is accompanied by additional resources, it can improve the quality of work and the quality of care, especially if it also promotes teamwork. In Norway, laundry work serves as an entry point for foreigners who did not pass the language test, giving them some opportunity to improve and putting them in a position to move to other work. We were told that the Norwegian workers at our site gave language classes to immigrant workers, teaching them not only about words but also about their meaning in this context. The teaching was done as part of the workday and provided shared experiences.

In sum, laundry and clothing help to illustrate how an increasingly flexible division of labour in nursing homes can mean more integrated care as well as more variety and autonomy for workers, which can benefit residents as well. However, if the main purpose is to cut jobs and if the strategy fails to take skills into account, the result can be the reverse.

SWITCHING IT UP: JOB ROTATION AND SHIFT WORK

Another way that laundry work can be reorganized in ways that expand the range of workers' tasks is through job rotation, shifting workers throughout the facility at a given time or on an as-needed basis. It was common for laundry workers in our study to have their job combined with housekeeping, either splitting their shifts between the two jobs as they did in BC or alternating positions as we saw in Nova Scotia. At sites in Ontario, it is housekeeping staff who remove soiled linen, return clean clothing to residents, and stock clean towels in residents' rooms at the start of the day. In a Norwegian home, housekeeping staff are reassigned to the laundry room on an as-needed basis. Elsewhere, housekeeping staff spoke to us of helping out in the laundry room when needed.

Laundry industry publications encourage nursing homes to implement such rotation systems between laundry and housekeeping departments as a way to promote workplace efficiency (Bowers et al. 2009; Williamson 2011). Labour costs are cited as being the biggest expense of an LTRC laundry service (Zimring 1998). Administrators are encouraged to find ways to reduce labour costs to optimize laundry according to principles of "maximum efficiency" (Zimring 1998) by streamlining labour processes to the bare minimum required, following practices in the for-profit sector. Cross-training workers in multiple jobs means they can be reassigned and shuffled about the facility according to staffing needs. Reassigning workers to departments where staffing is short allows a facility to continue operating under perpetually short-staffed conditions. A nursing home manager in BC described their facility's method of rotating a cleaner onto laundry duty at a certain time in the day, as this provided an extra part-time worker for the in-house laundry department where the workload is "very heavy duty." By rotating cleaning staff into laundry, management is able to avoid hiring additional laundry staff, keeping labour costs down. In effect, this strategy means that workers are required to be more flexible in the range of jobs they can perform (Coyle 2005).

This approach to work organization can be quite problematic from the perspective of the workers. One cleaner at an Ontario facility that had recently implemented a job rotation system for cleaning and laundry departments spoke at length of dreading her eventual return to the laundry, as laundry work required skills she did not have while ignoring the skills she does have: "It's a rotation so I will be going into the laundry in October and I am going to do that. And I'm good at what I do, housekeeping, but they are telling me I'm not good in English. But spelling, if I have to look at the names hanging up, I have to match the names, like the alphabet, because I'm not good at that. But they know that. Still they are sending me. I'll be behind … They don't realize people apply for a certain job because they are good at it. But they are throwing us in [the laundry]." As a result of this rotation system, this cleaner told us that she no longer feels valued at her job.

This rotation also requires a change to evening work shifts, causing difficulties as another cleaner explained because, like most women, she has additional care responsibilities at home: "We were hired for morning shift, but now they are throwing us in the evening shift [when rotating to laundry]. With me, my place, I have parents with me, and my dad has dementia. I take care of him in the night. So when this [rotation] happens it's going to be hard. So my flexibility will be very, very bad. But I have no choice."

This kind of rotation did not create greater variety in tasks. Indeed it meant the opposite. Before this new work organization, "the nursing staff used to make two beds or three beds for a day. Now we have to make twenty-five beds for a day, for that evening, in two and a half hours. In two and a half hours they have to make them. And in a six-month period we actually make 8,800 beds. You really hurt yourself. But it doesn't bother [the management]. It doesn't bother them. That is what I feel sad. Very sad … You have no choice." In order to keep her cleaning job, this worker must endure a mandatory rotation into the laundry department. Cleaners at this facility also spoke of their worry that laundry workers, when rotating into their cleaning positions from the comparative isolation of the laundry department, would not know the residents well enough to be able to return clothing, leading to more mistakes and lost items. Here, rotating workers between cleaning and laundry appears to have been problematic for worker well-being and morale, with additional negative consequences for the care of residents' clothing.

Rotating workers between different kinds of work is recommended in the industry literature as a way of preventing staff from becoming bored (Shady 2004), and thereby less productive, when they perform the same repetitive and monotonous tasks. Some workers, like a Nova Scotia cleaner/laundry worker we talked with, saw this work switching as beneficial. It allowed for some variety in the job and a chance to get out of the laundry room. Others saw this switching as a way to increase their workloads without giving them more time or more pay.

Shift work and the use of part-time and casual labour is another way that the labour of laundry can be divided up. Nursing homes need to bring in people when staff have holidays or take sick leave, and some women especially prefer part-time work given their additional responsibilities for care in their own homes. A UK laundry worker explained that she started part-time when "my kids were a lot younger so it had to be these hours ... and I could only come in some days. And they agreed to that so I thought, well, I'm not going to get a better job than that. So it just carried on and they kept phoning me to see if I was free when they were short-staffed. So yeah. We've got quite a few banked people, haven't we?" It worked for her in part because the home provided training and the opportunity to move into full-time when her responsibilities for childcare declined. Such a shift can be supported by law. For example, a worker in Norway reported, "there is also a law that states that anyone who works for the City of Oslo for ten years [is] supposed to be given permanent positions." Permanent part-time employees, as we saw in Manitoba, can develop relationships with others on the care team and with residents in ways that enhance the overall work process.

Issues arise, however, when part-time or casual workers are brought in who have no permanent ties to or experience in the nursing home. Temporary part-time and casual workers can mean more work for the permanent staff and lost clothes for residents, as an interview with two care workers from Ontario illustrates: "Sometimes during the days when we change their clothes, you know, and then some other clothes is mixed. That's the big problem for us too. We're getting the clothes. 'Oh, this is not for her. This is for the other.' I don't know why that is happening because we sorted out already ... Because there's names on the wall and there's names on the clothes. So why is her clothes down the hall and three doors down? Well, that's people that's part-time and they are casual and they get it mixed up." Most part-time and casual workers do not know residents as well as the full-time permanent staff, and have trouble returning clean clothing.

In sum, expanding jobs can mean more integrated care as well as more variety and autonomy for workers. A more flexible division of labour can benefit residents as well. However, if the main purpose is to cut jobs and if the strategy fails to take skills into account, the result can be the reverse. Similarly, as these experiences with laundry illustrate, part-time and casual employment can have its benefits, but only if there are real options and supports.

UNPAID WORK ORGANIZATION: FILLING IN FOR GAPS IN CARE

It is not only the paid staff who do the clothes and laundry work. Families, friends, relatives, and volunteers all play a part and that part is growing, often in ways that can mean additional pressures on the paid staff at the same time as it reduces other aspects of their work. Moreover, paid staff often take on additional unpaid work as a way of filling gaps in care when other unpaid workers are not available, or when the care is insufficient to meet residents' needs. Examining the who, why, and how of unpaid labour helps to reveal gaps and inadequacies in nursing home care, underlying assumptions about responsibility for care, and problems with too-narrow definitions of what is needed for care. This examination also reveals what is specific about the division of labour in nursing homes, given that unpaid labour is assumed to be part of the work organization.

Family members of residents are the most common source of unpaid labour in nursing homes, and for some family members, laundry and clothing is an area of ongoing involvement in their relative's nursing home life. The work of selecting the clothing to take to the home most often falls to them, with the selection based on cultural values as well as on instructions from the nursing home and on ideas about what kinds of clothes are suitable for the setting, for the resident, and for laundry in the home. In a Manitoba home, the handbook informs residents and their relatives that clothing must be "comfortable and easy to put on and take off," a common recommendation in the homes we visited. All personal clothing has to be labelled, even if the family intends to take responsibility for cleaning. The very act of labelling can be a reminder of the loss of a life lived independently outside of facility-based care, and it is no guarantee that clothes will not be lost in the laundry process or lost to other residents who wander into private rooms or who intervene in the nursing home's laundry process.

All these factors influence what clothes residents have to wear. As one daughter of a resident told us, "of course, I have to make sure it's not something they can shrink. You know, it can be dried" – referring to clothing that can withstand the nursing home's drying machines. At a German nursing home, family members are warned through an information sheet not to bring in delicate items like woollen underwear, as underwear at this home is washed off-site at a commercial laundry where the machinery and temperatures will destroy wool items.

For many family members, the clothes work does not stop after selecting and providing clothing for nursing home admission (Keefe and Fancey 2000). Relatives frequently take on the laundry work themselves, at least in North America. A common reason we heard for doing so is dissatisfaction with the laundry services provided by the nursing home. For instance, we were told that family members washed their relatives' clothing themselves because items frequently went missing in nursing homes with fully outsourced laundry services and because the commercial machines used by laundry services have ruined sensitive fabrics. Another reason is that nursing home admission guidelines usually advise relatives and friends to take responsibility for any clothing that requires gentle care. More than one home asks families to provide a special container for such clothing and to "collect the laundry weekly."* Nursing homes may encour-

---

*Quoted from a Canadian nursing home's guidelines; further information cannot be provided in order to maintain anonymity.

age family members to do residents' laundry by installing on-site laundry machines for relatives to use, thus lowering the workloads of paid staff (Milch 1995), and associated labour costs.

Even at nursing homes where personal laundry is carried out in-house, family members still reported taking on laundering – for example, when temperatures are set too high for wool sweaters. At another BC-based facility with in-house laundry, a manager noted that it was actually better when family members do the laundry for residents, because "otherwise you have a lot of headaches" with family dissatisfaction. Family members also step in when a resident's individual needs cannot be adequately met by the nursing home laundry. For instance, a relative reported doing all of a resident's personal laundry at home, as the resident was allergic to the facility's laundry detergent. This particular Manitoba nursing home has done many things to address problems with the laundry. All clothing is washed in-house and missing items are reportedly a very rare problem, because the facility employs only one laundry worker who has come to know all the residents as she both picks up and delivers their clothes to their room. As a result, she knows the owner of each item. This site also has smaller washing units that are capable of handling more delicate items to avoid ruining clothing through unnecessarily high temperatures.

However, there are clearly limits to the ability of this laundry service to accommodate individual residents' needs. When we asked the laundry worker at this nursing home if it would be possible for family members to bring in their own detergent for her to use, she laughed and explained that this would be asking "a little too much" of her workload – unsurprising given that there is only one laundry worker for the whole facility. As these examples illustrate, the distinction between institutional and home-based care is thus somewhat false, as the contributions of family members support and sustain nursing home care when it is insufficient or inadequate. In this sense, the labour of family members serves to subsidize nursing home care, filling in the gaps in residents' care.

Conversely, some family members reported they had a hard time saving personal laundry from the nursing home's industrial process. At a residents' council meeting, a woman explained to us that daughters in her Asian culture are expected to do this work, and so she takes her mother's laundry home and washes it herself. However, she also described the multiple strategies she used to ensure that her mother's clothes were not taken away and destroyed in the laundry process. She saw care aides so stressed and so focused on getting tasks done that "they acted like robots," automatically picking up the clothes regardless of the signs she put on the clothes closet and the seals she put on laundry baskets.

This woman's experience, along with others, highlights how the terms "family" and "relative" obscure the profoundly gendered nature of this particular contribution to nursing home care. We found that most often the relatives who take on laundry for residents are women: wives, daughters, and granddaughters of residents who would bring laundry home or wash it for residents at on-site laundry rooms. In other words, it is mainly women who are filling in the gaps by taking on their relatives' laundry after nursing home admission. Women's involvement in laundry reflects a continuation of the gendered division of labour in the domestic sphere, as laundry is a part of the unpaid and invisible care labour that supports and sustains the private household (Armstrong and Kitts 2004). This gendered division of labour has also historically been sustained by the organization of paid labour around a male breadwinner model (Neysmith 1991; Knijn and Kremer 1997), a model that both assumes and relies upon unpaid domestic labour in the private sphere to provide the necessary care work of a household. The model may be outdated and there are shifts in what women and men do in the private home, but old patterns persist to some degree, especially among those now in nursing homes. To the extent that there are gaps in nursing home care that are filled by the ongoing work of family members, our observations with laundry and clothing demonstrate that this labour is distinctly gendered.

This unpaid labour is a resource that is not evenly distributed among nursing home residents. Making sure that residents have enough clothing costs money, and shopping for clothing takes time and requires one to be able to get to a store, purchase suitable clothing, and transport the clothing to the nursing home. Washing clothing in the home also takes time, money, a means of transporting clothing to and from the nursing home, the physical ability to lift loads of clothing into and out of machinery, and access to washing and drying machines to begin with. This means that there are many nursing home residents who do not have access to the unpaid labour of family members to assist with clothing and laundry. One Canadian wife of a resident explained to us the disparity this can create between residents:

> Well, one of the things that bothers me a great deal is the laundry. They dump everything together I guess in some kind of a very strong solution. Not only that, they rip perfectly good new shirts, for instance, or pants. They rip things and I think they need someone at least part-time to be here to repair the damage they do. I used to sew but I don't have my equipment here at all. Anyway, most people I think take the clothing home and do it but since I live in an apartment it costs a lot to wash and dry and I don't think I'd have the strength to continuously do his laundry. They've ruined quite a few of his shirts and I don't think that's fair.

The interview reveals two important issues with laundry work. First, replacing ruined clothing is costly, but as this excerpt illustrates, so too is washing laundry in the home. For residents who do not have family members who can make up for inadequacies with the laundry, ruined clothing can reinforce class differences between residents in a highly visible way. This has implications for both resident dignity and comfort. When family members are unable to make up for inadequate laundry care, residents may have to wear damaged or stained clothing, and clothes that can withstand the industrial treatment may not meet residents' preferences for how clothes look, feel, or make them feel. Second, the interview reveals the complicated nature of the work in nursing homes. Families cannot be counted on to do the work, although they often do it. Families also have a great deal to say about how the work is done, and workers often are the ones on the frontline who face the anger and pressure from families when clothes are lost, ruined, or dirty.

We found that in instances where family was not available to fill the gaps in residents' laundry/clothing needs, it is often the workers who take on the task. This usually entails going beyond the formal job descriptions, work organization, and/or rules of their workplace. For example, one Ontario resident told us about assistive personnel stepping outside of their formal job descriptions and taking on her personal laundry during their work shifts, rather than sending the clothing to the facility's outsourced laundry service. This resident's clothing had gone missing in the past, and in the absence of family members who can do the laundry for her, care workers addressed the problem by squeezing the resident's laundry into their daily workload. Amidst an overwhelming workload and insufficient laundry staffing for ironing to be included as a regular part of the laundry process, a laundry worker in a Nova Scotia nursing home explained that she works outside the boundaries of her own paid schedule to make sure that residents' clothes are ironed, as for her this is an important element in providing good-quality care. Similarly, an Ontario cleaner spoke to us about sorting out residents' clothing in their drawers, organizing the contents by clothing type so that care workers would have an easier time when dressing residents. As she explained, care workers "only have an hour to do whatever they have to do," so sorting the clothing is an important way of giving care workers a bit more time to perform daily care, which includes dressing residents for the day. It should be noted that in a Swedish home we visited, workers were paid for such tasks.

As these experiences with laundry and clothing illustrate, the unpaid labour of paid nursing home staff can take many forms. Such labour can be thought of as strategies developed by workers in order to meet residents' needs despite insufficient nursing home resources (Armstrong et al. 2009). The fact that this labour takes place outside of the formal organization of work points to a too-narrow definition of what kind and amount of labour is needed for nursing home care, and a failure to fully incorporate clothing and laundry as a critical element of care. Workers have to work around and beyond their job descriptions and shift timing in order to meet adequately residents' clothing and laundry needs. These workaround strategies can be understood as "responses to structural/political conditions that render staff unable to produce adequate care to meet the needs of a resident" (DeForge et al. 2011, 424). Our research indicates these conditions include too little time, too few staff, and an outsourced laundry service that loses or destroys residents' clothing. And in the context of care work, it is women who are most likely to feel compelled to contribute their own time, energy, and/or resources to make up the difference, as Baines's (2004; 2006) research illustrates.

At times workers' unpaid labour may also involve working around the nursing home rules. Assistive personnel at one facility answered the question "what makes you feel bad when you're done your work day?" by explaining how they broke the rules to make sure that residents have something suitable to wear: "You want to dress the patient and they got rags. They don't have any visitors. So it's us who try to get some nicer clothes. But you have to run to get these clothes. If you don't care what the look of your patient is, you're going to put the rags on. If you don't want them to look like this, you're going to run. You're going to spend time." Asked if there are extra clothes, the worker responds, "We build that too … It's our store … And we're not supposed to do it." They had a strategy for getting the clothes for their store. "If someone passed away we would keep the good clothes and we marked them [with new names], but then they said, 'No, you can't do that anymore.'" According to the workers, they were told to stop because the centralized laundry did not want to do the work of changing the names and some families objected. But "we know some family would not put these clothes on, but some people, you know, they don't have any visitors. Nobody there for them. Sometimes you're the only ones taking care of them." They "spend time" and "run" to make this happen, in order to avoid residents being dressed in substandard clothing.

This example points to two issues in the care of residents' clothing. First, there is an implicit assumption built into the operations of at least the North American nursing homes that family members are primarily responsible for making sure that residents have enough clothing – the assumption, in other words, that family will be able to be there to meet the residents' needs. When residents have "nobody there for them" to take on this work, it falls to care staff to devise strategies to ensure that residents have sufficient clothing. They do so in ways that usually go beyond their job descriptions. These workers' experiences demonstrate how assistive personnel additionally provide unpaid and unrecognized labour in order to compensate for inadequacies in care (Baines 2004; 2006) – in this instance, the absence of family members to provide sufficient and appropriate clothing.

Second, the effort of care workers to arrange a supply of extra clothing reveals that the definition of nursing home resident care needs fails to account fully for all the necessary elements of residents' care. As Day (2014) has argued, the daily/nightly scramble of direct care workers to "make it work" must be contextualized by the failure of policy, regulations, and long-term care funding to account for the full range of residents' daily care needs. Laundry and clothing care are increasingly understood as ancillary to care, defined out of the care of nursing homes, and reclassified as "hotel" services rather than as integral to care work (Cohen 2001). Furthermore, standardized measurements used to assess and plan for nursing home residents' care tend to focus on their physical conditions and medical needs, and hence cannot capture inequality among residents in terms of available resources or informal support (Kontos, Miller, and Mitchell 2010). Workers' experiences with laundry labour thus reveal the implications – not only for residents, but also for workers – of defining care needs too narrowly.

LESSONS LEARNED IN LAUNDRY/CLOTHING WORK

In its association with home, domesticity, and the role of women, the labour involved in laundry and clothing is often invisible (van Herk 2002). From the perspective of feminist political economy, examining this invisible labour offers some important lessons about the organization of nursing home work more broadly, and its consequences for workers, residents, and their families.

Two broad approaches to the organization of care work are evident in the nursing homes we visited, each of which stems from particular notions about the work and about workers. As work that is often considered marginal to care, laundry and clothing illustrate hierarchical boundaries in the detailed division of nursing home labour and the ways that the organization of nursing home work is gendered, racialized, and classed. Laundry and clothing are the work of those who clean the bodies and physical spaces of the nursing home: workers who are lowest on the care work hierarchy, are most often women, and are increasingly drawn from racialized/immigrant communities. Such a division is supported by medical approaches that give priority to clinical care and fits with neo-liberal market approaches to work organization. It has also been supported by many workers' organizations as a way of ensuring skilled care, while it has not often been opposed by those whose jobs have been defined as unskilled. Instead, these worker organizations have focused on protecting pay, benefits, security, and working conditions, all of which are under threat in neo-liberalism.

A second approach in neo-liberalism is the reorganization of care work to expand workers' job descriptions through an increasingly flexible division of labour. Although it can lead to more integrated care, more teamwork, and more autonomy for workers, under market-based principles this reorganization can have significant negative consequences in assuming that the workloads of those defined as unskilled can be endlessly extended and that workers can be endlessly flexible in the tasks they perform.

Both approaches assume some unpaid work. Most often this work is done by female relatives. Doing laundry for their relative can be an important source of participation for these women, a way to help their relative and improve their well-being (Habjanic and Pajkinhar 2013). But it can also make life difficult for the many women with paid employment or for those without transport or access to washing machines. In the absence of families or when they fail to take on the job, the paid staff often step in to fill the gaps. We saw examples in Sweden where this gap work was paid in the form of banked work hours, but such compensation was not evident in the UK or North America.

Laundry and clothing simultaneously illustrate where the boundaries lie in nursing home work and the complex as well as the diverse divisions of labour in nursing home care. These complexities became evident in our site visits both within and across jurisdictions. It also became evident that the form of work organization alone does not create conditions that allow meaningful labour and relational care. Adequate staff and services united under one employer are necessary, whatever the division of labour. Without adequate staff and with services contracted out, the flexible division of labour that contributes to more integrated care and teamwork is undermined. The flexible division of labour in a Swedish facility is strained when tasks are added in order to reduce staff. Regulations are also a critical factor. Because the regulations do not require everyone at the table by a set time, the Nova Scotia workers can get residents up at the pace preferred by residents and at a pace that allows workers not only to balance tasks but also to chat. The physical environment and equipment can structure laundry work organization too. In one Swedish home with washing machines in every room, it makes sense for the person also providing personal care to do the laundry. In contrast, machines in the basement in a Canadian home isolated the laundry worker from residents.

Managerial approaches to work organization also matter. Based on a new model of care, a UK manager resisted regulations and historical practices that narrowly defined tasks, while a new building allowed a creative Manitoba manager to hire the staff and train them all to work with residents. Government policies on both licensing occupations and education, along with union efforts to protect workers, shape the extent to which work can be flexible and recognized as skilled. On the one hand, the unions and government policies in Canada help ensure safe care by defining scope of practice, but on the other, they contribute to rigid work hierarchies. Similarly, government efforts intended to ensure safety through auditing can reinforce hierarchies that make it more difficult to provide integrated care or work in teams, as we saw in Ontario. Union contracts can also protect part-time workers not only by ensuring they have appropriate pay and benefits but also by providing job security that can ensure continuity in care, and by limiting the hiring of casual workers as we saw in Manitoba. They can also support movement into other positions, as we saw in Norway. Finally, formal training and the recognition of informal learning can help address the notion that clothes and laundry work is unskilled labour any woman can do because she is a woman.

Building on this analysis, we now turn to examine a further contextual layer that affects the experience of laundry work and care: the working conditions and risks associated with this labour.

3

Risky Business

Work is often dangerous to the health of those who do it and to the health of those for whom the work is done. The work of laundry and clothing is no exception. Indeed, in Canada, absenteeism as a result of injury and illness is twice as high for workers in assisting occupations as it is for other health care workers, although rates are lower in other countries such as Sweden (Armstrong and Laxer 2012). The risks and how they are addressed are shaped by notions about the nature of the job, about gender, about efficiency, about cost, and about care. In this chapter, we examine how these forces frame both the recognized and unrecognized risks of laundry and clothing work in nursing homes and their consequences not only for those who live and work there but for those outside the home as well.

We begin this chapter by exploring the recognized links between the work and healthy environments. Laundry is an important part of managing risks to resident health, and this shapes how laundry workers are trained and how laundry work is organized. As laundry is crucial for maintaining sanitary conditions, laundry workers are "on the front lines when it comes to safe-guarding long-term care residents' health, cleanliness and quality of life" (Andrews 2013, 28). Effectively and efficiently managing risks to residents is part of a broader focus on accountability in nursing home care – primarily in terms of being accountable for residents' physical health. However, what is often missing from strategies for managing laundry as a health risk is an understanding of how laundry working conditions contribute to the effectiveness of infection control, to worker health, and to resident comfort as well as to their dignity. Workers' ability to manage health risks for residents and for themselves depends on having the appropriate equipment and training, so processes of cost-cutting, downsizing, and outsourcing the laundry all have implications for resident health. Thus, while the role of laundry in maintaining healthy environments is widely acknowledged, efforts to ensure a healthy environment are often undermined by a failure to recognize what other kinds of conditions are necessary for the health and well-being of residents and workers. Meanwhile, the work related to clothing has few recognized risks, and those that are recognized may be dismissed as necessary parts of the work.

We then turn to examine risks that frequently go unrecognized. As Messing (1997; 1998a) has argued, the occupational hazards of jobs traditionally occupied by women such as cleaning, care work, and laundry work have been largely neglected compared with those of traditionally male occupations such as those in construction, which are more often studied and readily recognized as dangerous. These differences in recognizing occupational hazards are rooted in assumptions about the nature of work and risks as well as about gender – integrated assumptions that have an impact on how risks are addressed (Campbell 2013).

One reason the hazards of laundry and clothing work may go unrecognized is its association with domestic labour. It is too often assumed that tasks associated with housework are neither dangerous nor demanding (Hall 1992; Rosenberg 1987). Moreover, because women do similar work at home, the health consequences of this type of paid job may be falsely attributed to their work at home, making it difficult for workers to obtain compensation for workplace injuries. Furthermore, given that male-dominated workplaces have been more frequently studied as dangerous, the models for what counts as a workplace hazard tend to fit better with work traditionally done by men. Male-dominated work thought of as hazardous is most often work characterized by obvious accidents and by accidents that are obviously the product of the work. As the European Agency for Safety and Health at Work (2003, 10) points out, "In general, men suffer more accidents and injuries at work than women do, whereas women report more health problems such as upper limb disorders and stress." With male workplaces as the standard, workplace hazards are frequently defined primarily as threats of immediate physical injury. This leaves out or underplays injuries that cannot be attributed to a single incident, such as pain, stress, strain, exhaustion, and sickness that build up over time. It also leaves out the consequences of workplace bullying, racism, violence, and harassment.

Finally, we look at strategies from governments, managers, and workers to address risks. Government employment regulations provide some protection to workers, although such regulations are not always effectively enforced (Vosko and Thomas 2014). Managerial approaches and unions also mitigate some of the obvious hazards. However, workers face a number of barriers to having the risks of their job acknowledged, due in large measure to perceptions about what counts as risky work and what counts as an injury, as well as to the tendency to neglect the underlying structural conditions that shape workplace hazards. These conditions contribute to one of the least visible risks of laundry and clothing work that we discuss in the section on unrecognized risks; namely, increasingly precarious labour. Recognizing that that the conditions of work are the conditions of care means recognizing that the well-being of workers and those for whom they care are inextricably linked.

THE RECOGNIZED RISKS

Whether or not risks are recognized depends on how risks are defined and identified. In terms of recognized risks, laundry is primarily approached as an aspect of infection control in health care settings. Like cleaning (Dancer 2009; Dancer 2011; Denton et al. 2004; Messing 1998b), laundry plays a significant role in maintaining healthy environments. Like hospital patients, nursing home residents have complex health needs that make them particularly vulnerable to infection. Unlike hospital patients, however, most residents have chronic illnesses and/or a level of frailty that mean they may live in the nursing home for a relatively long time. This makes them particularly vulnerable to problems such as bedsores that can be affected by how and how often the linens are washed. Furthermore, residents in nursing homes wear their own clothes, making hospital infection control approaches more difficult in the absence of easily sanitized hospital gowns.

From a public health perspective, laundry is recognized as a source of potential environmental contamination (Barrie et al. 1994; Chau et al. 2010; CUPE 2003; Greig and Lee 2009). Indeed, substantial evidence from hospitals shows that proper attention to sanitary laundry processing is important for infection control (Barrie 1994; Chau et al. 2010; Balm et al. 2012; Duffy et al. 2014; Fijan, Sostar-Turk, and Cencic 2005) and this research is reflected in quality indicators. Given the risks measured by quality indicators, recognized laundry risks tend to be related to the processes and equipment for maintaining sanitary conditions and preventing the spread of infections (Greig and Lee 2009).

Potential risks in laundry work documented in the literature include exposure to hazardous material encountered in the laundry, exposure to dangerous chemicals, and unsafe working conditions such as hot and humid laundry rooms (Thielen 2003). Much of this research has been conducted in commercial or hospital laundries. It is, however, important to distinguish laundry work in health care settings from laundry work in other settings, not only in terms of the risks to workers' health and well-being but also in terms of the skills and strategies required to navigate these risks. Laundry workers in all health care settings face unique on-the-job dangers, such as injury from needles concealed in the laundry (Shiao et al. 2001; Smith 2003). Laundry workers are not only at risk of infection due to handling contaminated laundry (Borg and Portelli 1999; Cohen 2001; Sepkowitz 1996; Standaert, Hutcheson, and Schaffner 1994); they are also at risk of injury due to prolonged exposure to the dangerous chemicals used to sanitize contaminated laundry in health care settings (Andrews 2011; Kovacs 2012). And laundry workers are additionally at risk outside the laundry room. Louther et al. (1997) report that, compared to all other occupational categories such as nursing, social services, and laboratory staff, it is hospital housekeeping staff – including laundry workers – who are at greatest risk for occupationally acquired tuberculosis. The authors suggest that airborne infections may not be seen as a risk for housekeeping staff, leading to more limited use of masks among these workers as they move throughout the building. These workers frequently also have less education on how to manage this risk relative to the nursing staff, raising a question about inequalities inherent to the division of labour and subsequent training.

In addition to these risks, however, nursing home workers face specific risks associated with laundry work. Residents wear their own clothes in nursing homes and incontinence is especially common in these settings, placing nursing home laundry workers at particular risk for infection as a condition of their work (Standaert, Hutcheson, and Schaffner 1994). Furthermore, personal clothes are harder to wash and it is much more difficult to detect hidden hazards in them compared to hospital gowns and sheets.

In the nursing homes of our study, we observed how the focus on particular kinds of health risks shapes the methods and equipment for collecting, transporting, and storing soiled laundry. While we turn to means of addressing health hazards in the second half of this chapter, it is worth noting here a couple of examples that illustrate the emphasis on infection containment. For instance, some homes had separate rooms for storing clean and soiled laundry to prevent cross-contamination. One home collected all laundry in disposable plastic bags rather than in reusable laundry bins in order to avoid contamination. In some homes, gloves were provided to laundry workers moving between rooms to gather soiled laundry. Workers in the laundry room at a UK home told us that wearing gloves was also important when sorting through the laundry as linen and clothes can be contaminated with infectious soiling and, in their words, "you never know what you're going to pick up" given the way that fabric can conceal soiling and hidden objects.

Sanitation concerns also dictate the washing process itself, including the temperature for washing laundry as well as the types of chemicals that are used in the wash. The chemicals required to remove all contaminants are both expensive and dangerous, a recognized hazard in many homes. As a regional vice-president for the US-based Healthcare Services Group explained, "These are industrial-strength chemicals and they have to be handled right, the formulas in the machines have to be right, and people have to be trained to use them in the machines. They must make sure linens are cleaned and sanitized and, more importantly, that whatever chemicals are used are thoroughly removed" (quoted in Andrews 2013). This kind of risk was recognized in many of the places we visited and was evident in the equipment. A maintenance worker at a Texas nursing home showed us the particularly high-tech washing machines in the laundry room of his home, which dispensed the precise amounts of chemical cleaners prescribed for sanitizing the laundry. Such automatic dispensers are common, allowing workers both to avoid touching the chemicals for each wash and to precisely measure them, thus controlling costs.

As the above quote indicates, concerns about the health risks of laundry also inform how laundry workers are trained, although training depends not only on what kinds of soiling are perceived as being hazardous but also, as we discuss in the previous chapter, on how laundry work is organized. For instance, at a UK nursing home we learned that designated laundry workers are trained in hygiene and infection control. In homes without designated laundry workers, however, this kind of training was less common. The training we did hear about was focused more on protecting the laundry than on protecting the laundry worker.

Although sanitation concerns often take primacy, other risks are also recognized to some extent. As is the case with all workplaces covered by government regulations and reflecting standards based on male-dominated workplaces, some physical injuries directly related to the work are recognized as a safety issue resulting from the job. Laundry work is very physically demanding labour (Gunnarsdóttir and Björnsdóttir 2003). Frequent bending, heavy loads, and poorly designed workstations that require awkward twisting, reaching, and bending can lead to strain and musculoskeletal injury among workers (Shady 2006; Andrews 2011; Sacouche, Morrone, and da Silva 2012; Wands and Yassi 1993), as can having improper equipment (Andrews 2009) or unnecessarily heavy supplies such as liquid detergent rather than powder (Maher 2001).

Acknowledging these hazards, a staff manual from one Canadian home we visited has pictures illustrating the physical risks associated with nursing home work. All but four of the fifteen pictures illustrating risks have men doing the work of lifting heavy boxes or gripping heavy tools. One woman is pictured pushing a cart of boxes, while the other women are answering the phone or working at a computer or a cash register. None include patients or depict laundry rooms. Yet laundry workers often lift heavy loads without the aid of the sorts of equipment pictured in the manual.

Furthermore, as we noted earlier, much of the work of clothing and laundry is done by other assistive personnel and it is usually done far away from a laundry room where safe equipment and safety rules are often in place. In addition to the physical lifting, this work is not without its own specific risks. Dressing and undressing, and especially changing diapers, expose workers to physical risks both because this is such intimate work and because workers are so close to the residents. We heard many reports, especially in North America, of residents lashing out when this clothing work was under way. Canadian workers told us they are exposed to "verbal and physical" abuse; they are "kicked, punched, spit [on], [bitten]." Workers showed us scratches that they had most frequently received when the more intimate bodily work such as dressing was being done. A male worker at one Ontario home came into an interview bleeding from his arm after a resident had scratched at him during care. Some workers understood dementia as the cause of this violence. Talking about the physical, but also verbal and sometimes racist abuse they face, it was common for Canadian workers to say something like, as one care worker put it, "we know that it's the illness that's progressing. It's not who they were before."

Here the line blurs between the recognized and unrecognized risks of laundry and clothing work. While there is a growing movement to recognize violence against health care workers that was evident in many signs we saw posted in nursing homes, workers frequently reported they were often told by management that that violence was a part of the job and thus not a basis for recognized injury. But others attributed the violence to lack of care, itself the product of low staffing and rushed procedures. The latter interpretation is supported by research. Residents are less likely to resist if they are treated with respect and in a caring way, resulting in less risk to the worker. But a rushed, stressed, disrespected worker is less likely to be able to treat residents with respect.

There is another important risk that is usually recognized: the risk of smells. Field notes from a Canadian site indicated that some places take the problem seriously:

There is no hospital smell at all. There was only a brief stinky smell but the PSW [personal support worker] removed it right away, and otherwise there's been nearly no smell, other than the resident's nice perfume when she came by! E. says right away that

yes, they try very hard to make sure if there's a smelly diaper to
remove it right away; she says that sometimes they will not keep it
in the hallway garbage cart but rather will put it in the utility
room garbage instead, this is how they try to keep things smelling
nice "because they don't want to be in that, and you don't want to
have to work in that."

However, at a site in Texas we visited as part of the site selection process,
the smell of urine permeated the entire nursing home and made
breathing hard even in the director's office. The smell was the main reason we rejected this place as a site to search for promising practices.

In sum, the recognized risks in laundry and clothing work tend to
be those associated with infection control or with the physical risks
often associated with men's work. But there are other risks we heard
about that were seldom recognized in the places we visited.

THE UNRECOGNIZED RISKS:
HAZARDOUS WORK AND WORKING CONDITIONS

Workplace injuries in women-dominated jobs – including nursing
home laundry and clothes work – do not fit within the standard accident or direct causal framework (Forastieri 2000; Messing et al. 2000).
When workers' illnesses and injuries fall outside of the accident
framework, they often face barriers to having these harms understood
as a product of their work environments. Moreover, injuries may not
be recognized as workplace hazards if the assumption is made that
workers can avoid such injuries – a problem often faced by care workers – or if it is assumed that the problem may arise from women's
unpaid work at home.

While the public health risks posed by laundry itself in terms of
infection control, sanitation, and exposure to chemicals are often recognized in both nursing home regulations and research literature, the
risks of laundry as work are far less often acknowledged. Much of
laundry and clothing work tends to fall outside of the dominant
understanding of what counts as dangerous work, based on the perception that women's work is "light," less physically demanding, and
less accident-prone (Messing 1997; 1998a). There is, however, substantial evidence that laundry work can be hazardous to health in ways

other than those discussed in the previous section. While there are some hazards that are a product of the work itself, hazardous conditions are further shaped by the particular way the work is organized, by workplace design, and by the kinds of equipment that workers have access to, as well as by how risk is understood.

Throughout the sites of our study we heard of workers being injured when lifting heavy bags of laundry for delivery to centralized laundry services and when pushing heavy linen carts around the carpeted residential floors. Laundry workers at multiple nursing homes experienced severe back pain and shoulder pain from lifting heavy weights and pulling laundry out of bins and machines, and painful repetitive strain injuries from performing the same motions over time. But while the potential injuries of this physically demanding job may be more readily recognized, the hazards in how the work is divided and allocated are a factor contributing to workers' pains and injuries that is less often acknowledged. Consider the following notes from a conversation with a woman in her late fifties, who vividly illustrated for us the toll that laundry work takes on the body at her Ontario nursing home:

> Our cleaner goes on to explain to me that she does hate one aspect of her job which is the laundry. She said she hates that job and the division of labour there and never wants to go back to do that job again. She put her hands together and looked skyward and said she prayed to God she would never have to go back there. When I asked her why, since this seemed fairly melodramatic, she said that the work load is way too heavy, it's the kind of work load that hurts your body so that you go home every night and you have an aching shoulder, you can barely move your arm and your back hurts. My shoulder is starting to hurt just listening to this story and the distress in her voice. She said she was seeing a physiotherapist, a chiropractor, she took anti-inflammatories, but she said she would wake up in the night with her arm completely stiffened to the point where she couldn't move it and her back so painful it woke her up.

This worker's concern was not only the work itself but also the fact that the work had recently been reorganized to include extra tasks, requiring workers to rush to get through the work of their shift as there was no increase in the laundry staffing levels following the change. Moreover, because this worker could not pinpoint a precise moment of injury in performing laundry work, she experienced difficulties in having her pain acknowledged and compensated by management.

The hazards of laundry labour related to work organization are not limited to the laundry room. Workers also spoke of strains and injuries in performing laundry-related tasks throughout the nursing home. At one Ontario nursing home, laundry workers explained that the most exhausting and painful aspect of their work actually takes place in residents' rooms: the daily job of stripping and making up beds. Changing the bed linen had previously been the responsibility of the nursing home's frontline care workers, with the work divided up so that each person had only a few beds to change per day. This task has now been reassigned to the facility's in-house laundry workers who, being far fewer in staffing numbers, must each strip and make up to twenty-five beds per day in order to keep up with the bed linen laundry schedule. The mattresses are thick and heavy, and the sheets must be firmly pulled and folded underneath each corner of the mattress, requiring each mattress to be lifted four times to make one bed. The sheer volume of beds in need of daily changing means that workers must move very fast to make sure that they get through the workload of their shift. As a result, they miss their breaks and risk not only exhaustion but also repetitive strain injuries in performing the same strenuous motions over and over within a condensed time-frame and without rest. Reassigning bed-making to laundry workers may have been a way to provide harried personal support workers with a little more time per shift to complete their own workloads, for as one laundry worker described it, the pace of direct care workers at this facility is "go, go, go, go." However, this change has clearly had reverberating negative consequences for the health and well-being of laundry workers to whom the task has fallen.

Poorly designed workplaces can also be harmful to the health of workers. Laundry room and process design are not only matters of efficiency but can jeopardize workers' health. Most of the in-house laundry rooms we observed were hot, crowded, very noisy, and often windowless rooms. At a Manitoba nursing home, the sole in-house laundry worker told us that, due to the windowless design of her laundry room, "if there was a fire outside my door, I would be finished because I have no escape." And dryers can put workers at risk of fire (Andrews 2013). At this same nursing home, the laundry room ventilation had to be sealed off as it was venting into the kitchen and spreading smells into the food preparation area, resulting in less air flow for the laundry workspace.

Design can have an impact on mental health as well. In nursing homes with centralized in-house laundry, the laundry department is typically located far from the residential floors, often in a basement. In these instances, laundry workers spoke to us about feeling isolated. Many worked alone, and those who had coworkers with them in the laundry room spoke of how lonely and boring their work would be without each other for company. For laundry work that is outsourced to off-site commercial laundry facilities, we can only guess at how far removed these workers may feel from the nursing home residents whose laundry they care for. Other laundry workers told us that changes to their working conditions such as expanding workloads, lower staffing levels, and rotation between cleaning and laundry departments have made them feel less valued and respected as members of the care team. The combination of physical isolation and occupying a low position on the care work hierarchy means that laundry workers are also often left out of nursing home celebrations and forgotten in shows of staff appreciation by family members. As one worker put it, relatives bring in treats for the nursing staff but "nothing ever comes downstairs to us cellar dwellers."

It has long been recognized that those with the least control in the workplace often experience the most stress (Karasek 1979). The feeling of being lowest in the care work hierarchy, and indeed excluded from the wider care work team, is particularly distressing for ancillary workers given that they take pride in their work as an important element in care (Messing 1998b). As one laundry worker in Ontario told us in response to being asked whether her work was valued in the nursing home, "you aren't so valued by the staff. But residents have always valued us." Furthermore, amidst the hierarchical ordering of nursing home work there is similarly a hierarchical ordering in the perception of dangerous work and working conditions. A laundry worker in Manitoba explained to us that "when it comes to safety and stuff like that … it's always the nurses [who] are thought of first, and then the health care aides, and then it's everybody else after that," referring to laundry workers as being last in line. While there is a tendency to lump together the various types of women's invisible labour in nursing homes, the visibility of workplace hazards appears to differ along the hierarchy of pay, professionalization, and perceived skill. That laundry workers feel their safety issues are less visible than those of nursing staff is particularly disconcerting given that care workers report facing significant barriers to having the hazards of their work acknowledged and addressed (Armstrong and Jansen 2000; Campbell 2013).

Discrimination and racism are also often hard to see and may be hidden by the composition of the workforce. Assistive personnel are disproportionately from racialized and/or immigrant communities and a growing number of them are men. The presence of male staff in homes mainly populated by female residents creates difficulties, we were told. We heard multiple reports in Canada of relatives refusing to have a man dress a female resident, in particular. One man on the family council of an Ontario nursing home told us that "no man will touch [his] wife." Given that most of these male workers are from racialized communities, it is hard to see to what extent such objections are mainly about race, but we also heard of instances when residents refused to be dressed by "that Black person." In some cases such objections were handled informally or formally by reorganizing the work, increasing the work for others and accepting the objections. It was justified to us on the grounds that residents were too old and/or demented to understand their racist comments. With little power and few credentials, more than one worker told us they have to "suck it up" because the managers side with the family.

Finally, precarity and marginalization can also make laundry and clothing work hazardous. Already marginalized older persons and persons from racialized/immigrant populations (Cohen and Cohen 2004; Laxer 2013) disproportionately do this work, and they can be further marginalized by precarity (Vosko 2006) and their location near the bottom of the health care hierarchy. As explored in chapter 1, in an industry where wages are already quite low regardless of ownership model, encroaching privatization has increasingly placed laundry workers at risk for job loss, poorer working conditions, and lower wages (Cohen and Cohen 2004; CUPE 2003; CUPE 2013; Grant, Pandey, and Townsend 2014; Pullen 2015; Rashid 2013; Stinson, Pollak, and Cohen 2005). The entire laundry department has been eliminated at some of the nursing homes in our study, with the work subsequently contracted out to private companies or downloaded onto care workers. Evidence from both Canada (McDonough 2000) and Europe (Ferrie et al. 2005; László et al. 2010) has demonstrated that job insecurity is associated with increased risk of poorer health, further challenging the notion that health care strategies can focus exclusively on training workers and providing protective gear. Moreover, research on dementia care indicates that continuity is critical to resident health, and knowledge about individual residents can help prevent violence (Bergland 2005), but precarity can make it difficult for workers to establish relationships with residents.

Laundry work can also be organized in ways that sustain workers' marginalization, such as requiring workers to work a very long time before they become eligible for pensions, or hiring workers on a part-time basis only. For instance, at a Norwegian nursing home in our study, the only permanent jobs available in the home were in frontline care work. However, to retain one's job as a care worker requires passing a standardized Norwegian language test. Workers who do not pass this test are transferred to the laundry/cleaning department, where work is part-time only, and where having Norwegian language skills is considered less important because they are not "client-facing." By implementing the language test as a condition of permanent work, employers retain a pool of cheap, marginalized, and precarious laundry/cleaning labour hired on a part-time basis and under part-time conditions. Furthermore, workers have few opportunities to improve their language skills in the relative isolation of the laundry department, preventing them from moving into more secure and better paying care work positions. It should be noted, however, that other workers have considerable job security and autonomy in the Norwegian homes we visited.

In one UK home we studied, the only full-time, permanent employees were the managers. The workers in this nursing home have what have come to be known as zero-hour contracts, which means the working hours are at the discretion of the employer (Government UK 2015). Workers are guaranteed only statutory annual leave and minimum wage, not sick pay. This workplace had a very flexible division of labour, and the precarious positions of the workers meant they had little option but to take on any tasks as requested if they wanted to get any hours, let alone full-time employment. While the workers we talked with did in general get the hours of paid work they wanted, there was a constant worry about whether or not they would have the hours they needed to survive. Here, too, there was a contrast with Sweden, where workers had considerable job security and were paid considerably above minimum wage – conditions that help them resist unsafe working conditions.

In short, those who do the laundry and clothing work face a wide range of risks to their health and well-being; however, these hazards often go unrecognized, pointing to the complexities of understanding the laundry and clothing work as risky. The fact that many workers experience non-physical harms suggests that injurious conditions are not exclusively due to excessive workloads or organization of the work. As Armstrong and Jansen (2000) have noted, additional factors such as the threat of job loss and conditions that damage workers' ability to feel their work is valued may compound the risk of ill health and well-being.

There are strategies in place to prevent injury and even to promote health. We have used some of these to illustrate the extent to which hazards are recognized. We now turn to examine in more detail government, managerial, and worker strategies that shape the context for health work and care.

GOVERNMENT STRATEGIES

Through policies, regulations, funding, and accountability measures, governments set many of the conditions for health and safety in these homes. All of the homes we visited receive some form of government funding and face accountability procedures. Even in Texas, where government regulation of workplaces is the most limited, we were repeatedly told that nursing homes are more regulated than the nuclear industry. All the homes we visited are subject to policies on health and safety, workers' compensation regulations, and reporting strategies, although there is significant variation among these policies and their enforcement in different jurisdictions. In all but Texas, unions also play a role. The processes reported in earlier sections of this chapter for handling chemicals are examples of labour standards in action. While it is not possible to explore all of these influences on risks to health in detail here, it is possible to highlight those we heard about in the sites we visited.

Most jurisdictions have workplace health and safety committees mandated by law. In Germany, for example, the law requires that all workplaces with more than twenty employees have occupational health and safety committees that include employees, that specialists in occupational health be available, and that paid sick leave be provided (WHO 2012, xiv). These committees, along with labour standards legislation, help provide some protection for the health of workers and address the absenteeism and turnover rates that cost both governments and individual employers (OECD 2011). While many of the strategies focus on the individual workers, some jurisdictions consider larger structural issues. According to the Organisation for Economic Co-operation and Development (2011, 202), "Countries with well-developed social dialogue and a structured approach to the recognition of worker's needs, such as the Netherlands, Norway, and Sweden, manage better retention than others with a limited development of structural dialogue."

The "structural dialogue" is supported by funding. Among the countries in our study, Norway and Sweden devote the most resources to long-term care while Canada devotes the least (OECD 2015, 209). The funds in Sweden and Norway contribute to higher staffing levels, which in turn help create safer conditions for both residents and workers. A comparative survey of nursing home workers in Nordic countries and Canada (Armstrong et al. 2009, figure 28) indicates that Canadian workers were more than six times as likely to report experiencing violence "more or less every day." At the same time, the Scandinavian workers were much less likely to say they had to leave essential work undone and much more likely to say they have the time to chat and provide other forms of social care. Their staffing levels are also much higher in comparison.

Such violence is increasingly recognized as a workplace hazard in long-term care, and many places we visited have official policies saying that violence is not acceptable. The Texas Department of Insurance, Division of Worker Compensation and Workplace Safety acknowledges that violence is a major issue for health care workers: "They are exposed to many safety and health hazards, including violence. Recent data indicate that hospital workers are at high risk for experiencing violence in the workplace. Several studies indicate that violence often takes place during times of high activity and interaction with patients, such as at meal times and during visiting hours and patient transportation. Assaults may occur when service is denied, when a patient is involuntarily admitted, or when a health care worker attempts to set limits on eating, drinking, or tobacco or alcohol use." However, all of the strategies suggested have to do with training individuals in how to handle potentially violent situations or with providing security measures such as locked doors. There is little recognition that adjusting working conditions, such as providing more staff with more regular shifts, would help prevent violence. Furthermore, there is no state policy in Texas requiring that workers receive sick leave or even reasonable vacations if they suffer from this violence.

Regulations that guide approaches to nursing home care also make a difference to violence levels. In a Nova Scotia home where residents can get up and have breakfast whenever they feel like it and where designated workers come in to serve breakfast, allowing care aides more time to dress residents, we heard much less about violence connected to clothes and the work of dressing residents. At other places in Canada, workers reported that rushing residents to get them up and dressed for breakfast often led to violent responses.

The absence of regulations also matters. While jurisdictions such as Ontario have detailed regulations about design features such as the size of windows in residents' rooms and about safety regulations such as fire escapes, there are fewer regulations about the design and location of laundry facilities. But the location and design of laundry rooms are important to the physical and mental health of laundry workers. The in-room washers and dryers that we observed in Scandinavian nursing homes mean workers spend very little time doing the laundry, handle lighter loads, and avoid the risks of cross-contamination. We observed a laundry room on the second floor of an assisted living facility that had large windows and great views, making a big difference in terms of the look of the workplace and the possibilities for light and air quality. The manager noted that the residents loved the room, making us wonder why governments do not consider such factors in regulating design.

There is a trend towards enhanced accountability to government through documentation evident in many of the jurisdictions in our study (Banerjee and Armstrong 2015; Lloyd et al. 2014). Recording the percentage of residents who contract new infections such as flu or bed sores (Berta et al. 2014) is just one example. This documentation can make threats to health more visible and contribute to higher, safer staffing levels that mean better health for residents and workers. For instance, recording the frequency of a resident's soiled laundry at a German nursing home in our study is used as a way to indicate the need for an upgraded level of care, as the manager explained to us (through a translator):

> TRANSLATOR: So you put your stick by the monitor and the care plan is shown, all the people there.
> INTERVIEWER: Every task is documented.
> TRANSLATOR: You just tap okay and with your signature it's signed that you have done these [tasks]. If there is something else to do like someone taken out the diaper and wet the bed, you washed the resident or changed the sheets and changed clothes, you could document this task also, additional.
> INTERVIEWER: And will it take it off the care plan for the next morning if that person needs to have a wash in the morning?
> TRANSLATOR: No, no. Just to see that you have done additional work. And if this gets common the care plan can be changed accordingly.
> INTERVIEWER: To another grade.
> TRANSLATOR: Yeah. There's more work. Hello health insurance. Look. This resident needs more care. Come on and check this and upgrade to the next level.

In this instance, the number of times a worker has had to change clothing or bedsheets is transformed into evidence of the need for an upgraded level of continence care. Documenting is important from an accountability perspective in reducing incidents of infection and, subsequently, in improving a nursing home's performance measures. But the German home has better funding and more staff compared to the US and Canada, which are also factors in these better performance results. Moreover, the reporting is directly linked to and results in more funding, with that money coming from health insurance. In Ontario, where accountability processes focus primarily on enhanced recording and reporting using specific, quantifiable performance measures, workers told us this meant increased time documenting but no more staff. The link between documenting and funding is quite weak. Funding is based primarily on three broad resident categories that are intended to reflect their overall needs, so the extra tasks resulting from a wet bed would not translate into more money. The result often is more pressure on both residents and workers, we were told.

Although workplace hazards may be recognized in the literature, there is no guarantee that these hazards will be acknowledged by government workplace compensation systems. The perception of what counts as an injury has implications for the ability to claim compensation and sick leave, especially for women (Lippel 2003). A laundry worker at a Manitoba nursing home told us about attempting to claim workers' compensation for a shoulder injury. As the sole laundry worker for the entire nursing home, she has experienced pain in her shoulder from daily hauling of wet and heavy loads of laundry. However, she told us her claim was dismissed because she couldn't "pinpoint" exactly how she was hurt in the course of her job. Asked if she had experienced any injuries, she said, "Just a shoulder and minor stuff." Asked if this injury was covered by workers' compensation, she responded that "they wouldn't because I couldn't pinpoint exactly how I hurt my shoulder. Like it has to be like I actually fell and hurt it right at that moment." In other words, this laundry worker was denied compensation for her injured shoulder as it was not a product of a single incident, such as a fall, but rather had built up over time. Her pain is minimized as just "minor stuff" because, in her words, "it's nothing that prevented me from moving," normalizing her experience and reflecting the notion that the only real or serious injury is a clearly identifiable incident resulting in incapacitation. In a job where the wear and tear on the body builds up over time, laundry workers may thus be particularly at risk of having their compensation claims dismissed and their injuries downplayed. Those injured while dressing residents face similar barriers, as we were told by a Nova Scotia worker who recounted her years of struggle to have her back problems compensated. She still goes in to work each day in pain.

Governments' adoption of market strategies, discussed in chapter 1, also shapes health and safety within long-term care. Support for contracting out services in BC, for example, is a critical factor in the precarity of the labour force in long-term care and thus a factor in health risk. So too is the failure to protect pay equity and other gains when jobs are moved or to promote job security for part-time employees. More casual and temporary part-time workers mean more people have to be trained about hazards at work, and their limited training can put permanent employees at risk.

In short, governments shape what employers can do and what they must do in terms of health and safety. Their influence goes well beyond setting rules for health and safety. Indeed, governments set the context for risks faced by both residents and staff. Nevertheless, managers still play a critical role.

MANAGERIAL STRATEGIES ADDRESSING RISKS

We saw a variety of managerial approaches to recognizing and addressing risks in the various homes we visited, ranging from a focus on individuals and accidents to larger structural strategies that had an impact on health. Most common were strategies to address the visible risks and the risks most often identified in health and safety standards, usually reflecting a focus on the medical and on the individual worker rather than on conditions of the work. In the case of less visible health hazards, there were fewer visible managerial strategies to address them.

In all the sites we visited, managers were very conscious of their staff illness and injury rates. All of them talked about developing the means to reduce these rates, but in North America and the UK especially they tended to focus on the individual rather than on systemic issues within the workplace. Similar to the recommendations for infection control, preventing injuries among laundry workers is often framed as a matter of providing workers with the right tools or training to get the job done safely, without addressing the specificities of laundry work. For instance, Fijan and Sostar-Turk (2012) recommend managing the risks of infection among hospital laundry workers by implementing guidelines for effective antimicrobial laundering as well as hygienic and common-sense processes such as handwashing. Other recommendations include education programs to improve proper disposal of medical sharps (Shiao et al. 2001), needle-searching machines to detect hidden sharps in the laundry (Smith 2003), and additional training and supervision of workers to ensure they do not fall into "bad habits" (Andrews 2011). Any or all of these can help reduce the spread of infection among residents and workers.

However, without strategies to recognize or alter laundry working conditions, the effectiveness of risk management strategies may be undermined. An example of the failure to recognize how the work is done comes from a UK nursing home. Laundry workers experiencing bad shoulder pains were given stools to sit on while pulling things out of the washing machine. But these stools were completely impractical for their work, as sitting does not allow for the substantial leverage needed to reach into the machine and pull out the wet, heavy loads of laundry. The stools went unused and workers' shoulder pain continued. While recommendations from the laundry literature include sorting laundry only after it is washed to avoid excessive handling and spread of infection (Ragone 2012), we found that workers are often required to sort laundry in its soiled state in order to appropriately customize the wash to fit different kinds of materials. This dilemma is exemplified particularly well at a Texas nursing home we visited, where care workers explained that laundry is sorted in order to be washed at different sites. Certain types of soiling, such as blood and bodily fluids other than urine, and communal supplies such as table cloths are sent to be washed separately by specialized on-site laundry workers who know (at least in theory) how to properly handle and clean these materials. While such a separation can ensure that the most dangerous laundry is subject to sanitary processing, the very act of sorting the dangerous from the not dangerous requires knowledge of the different kinds of health hazards. And many of the places we visited had no space to sort the laundry.

The literature also recommends that workers wear protective gear not only when handling dirty laundry but also when handling clean laundry to prevent cross-contamination (Gaubert 2010). Workers often have too little time or space to put on gloves and to wear masks when they switch from dirty to clean laundry or when they handle either of them. This is especially the case for assistive personnel who do a range of tasks in addition to dressing, undressing, and changing residents out of soiled clothing. In other words, just because safety equipment is made available does not mean that it will be used, or that the conditions of the workplace are conducive to their use. Masks to protect workers against chemicals and airborne contaminants may be extremely uncomfortable to wear in hot and stuffy laundry rooms, and gloves to protect against contamination and sharps injuries may make it harder for workers to grasp wet laundry (Kumar, Goud, and Joseph 2014). Safety equipment that gets in the way of workers' ability to do their job is far less likely to be used, especially where there is an emphasis on speed. It does, however, give the appearance of having accounted for occupational health and safety, and as such it places responsibility for injuries squarely onto workers.

Simply making safety equipment available to workers is insufficient unless the working conditions are conducive to sanitary laundry practices, and may work to absolve managers from responsibility for preventing health risks. It is thus important to begin from workers' experiences when addressing the safety of their working conditions, observing their work and involving them in the process of dealing with the risks that result from particular work processes and workplace design (Gunnarsdóttir and Björnsdóttir 2003; Sacouche, Morrone, and da Silva 2012). As the vice-president of a large US company providing services to health facilities puts it: "No one would willingly put people in danger, but if safety committees were more active, it would go a long way toward better resident protection and laundry and housekeeping should definitely be a part of that group" (quoted in Andrews 2013). In Sweden, we did see the entire range of workers participating on a daily basis on issues that included health, and doing so in ways that recognize multiple hazards.

Without such consultation, managers may fail to address underlying working conditions and work organization as a context for potential harm, even when attempting to take injury prevention seriously. For instance, at one Ontario nursing home the management complained that workers were filling bags of laundry too full, creating loads of laundry that were too heavy to lift and thus placing workers at risk for injury each time they lifted a bag. Adding a fill-to line on the bag did not address the problem. Workers continued filling the bag to maximum capacity, as this was a way to save some time by reducing the need to frequently empty the laundry bags. Rather than addressing the fact that workers had too little time to empty the laundry collection bags at a safer weight, management at this facility instead changed the size of the bags so that workers would be forced to empty them more frequently. While this addressed the problem of lifting heavy loads and prevented back strain, it did not address the underlying problem that workers have to rush to get through their workloads.

Similarly, many nursing homes have separate rooms for storing clean and dirty laundry to avoid cross-contamination, but the laundry collection process can undermine efforts to ensure sanitation in the laundry room. While centralized utility rooms for storing clean and dirty linen may help to avoid cross-contamination, this design can require workers to make frequent and often long-distance trips between residents' rooms and the utility room. A laundry worker in Manitoba explained how frustrating this process can be as a result of the facility design: "If I'm down at one end, I've got to run to the other end [to drop off soiled linen] and then I've got to run back to that end after I've washed my hands to pick up the clean stuff to run back to that end to make a bed." Designed with sanitation in mind, the location of utility rooms in this home clearly does not reflect the work processes of nursing home care, nor the working conditions that require workers to run to get through their workloads. The running can result in exhaustion and in avoidance of health protection strategies.

We also heard about managers who failed to recognize the link between injuries and the workplace, perhaps because of concern about having too many injuries on their records and about staffing in workers' absence. More than one manager told us that they were suspicious about requests for sick leave when an injury does not fit the "accident" framework. This was illustrated quite bluntly by one support services manager at a BC nursing home, who spoke of the need to be vigilant in preventing "abuse" of sick leave by support service staff who are simply "not happy at work" or are "lazy." In being prone to injuries that do not fit within the acceptable incident/accident framework, laundry and assistive personnel risk having their sick leave or injury deemed illegitimate, understood as a product of an individual's poor work ethic rather than working conditions.

We did, however, also hear about managers who recognized and acted on hazards. In a UK home, the manager made it very clear that she would not tolerate racist remarks or requests for changes based on racism. She told a family they would have to remove the resident if they refused care based on a worker's gender or race. We also saw other strategies to overcome the objections. In one case, a male worker was introduced by a woman who worked alongside the man to dress and bathe the residents until the resident became accustomed to his presence and would accept his care. In a Texas home, laundries on each floor reduced the need to take soiled laundry long distances, and the laundry was collected in sealed bags in each room to prevent smells as well as heavy loads.

These risk management efforts speak to the recognition that laundry is linked to the health of residents and the cleanliness of the nursing home environment. However, there are many ways that the effectiveness of nursing homes' approaches to risk management may be compromised by other aspects of work organization and time pressures. They can also be compromised by cost-cutting strategies taken from the for-profit sector. Despite the concern for infection control and accountability in nursing home settings, in several homes the link between laundry and health was insufficient to save the laundry department from being one of the first areas to experience budget cuts, downsizing, and outsourcing in the name of enhanced efficiencies. As with housekeeping budget cuts in health care settings (Armstrong et al. 2008; Armstrong and Armstrong 2010), cost-cutting in the laundry department has implications for the health and well-being of both residents and workers at risk. As one manager at an Ontario nursing home admitted, laundry services have a finite budget, so "you have to watch in terms of resident care and safety of the household."

The consequences of cost-cutting were evident to housekeeping workers we interviewed in Manitoba, who spoke of the implications for resident well-being and nursing home cleanliness when laundry budgets were cut. Audits of "inefficiencies" in the nursing home concluded that rubber draw sheets used on residents' beds were too expensive and unnecessary. They were subsequently eliminated. However, for workers this means that the entire bed now has to be changed when a resident is incontinent, which also often requires getting the resident up and out of bed in the night while all the bedding is changed. This increase in the amount of dirty laundry has also been accompanied by cuts to laundry staff. As a result, laundry is increasingly "piling up" in the nursing home, which additionally affects how the home smells. While eliminating rubber draw sheets has reduced some costs for the nursing home, residents are now up more at night, the volume of soiled laundry has increased, and the cleanliness of the nursing home environment has suffered considerably. This approach may be "efficient" from a particular cost perspective, but is clearly not effective for managing risks to residents' health.

Widespread cuts to laundry budgets mean fewer staff available to do the work or, as we noted in the previous chapter, the work is simply added to the workload of others. Remaining workers are rushed to get through their workload, leading to mistakes and corner-cutting that can endanger residents as well as workers. Such staff reductions often accompany the contracting out of services, as we explored in chapter 1. As with cleaning (Dryden and Stanford 2012), outsourcing the work also means that nursing homes have less control over the laundry process and less ability to monitor and correct for quality issues in ways that could increase efficiency. For example, in some homes where laundry is collected for washing in centralized facilities or for delivery to outsourced, off-site services, we saw large, open bags of soiled laundry crowded into hallways and left for hours, as laundry pickup occurs only at times designated by the contracting company. The smell alone was a hazard to the health and comfort of residents as well as to workers and visitors, and indicated the possibility of airborne contaminants. Residents and relatives may not have the ability to monitor the bacterial content of the linen and clothing, but they can tell when standards slip. We were told by relatives in a BC nursing home that cleanliness was noticeably worse after housekeeping services, including laundry, were outsourced. Privatization is also associated with less training and higher levels of turnover, further jeopardizing infection control as workers have fewer opportunities to learn the specialized skills required to ensure healthy environments (CUPE 2009).

In sum, managers do address some health issues for workers in ways that in turn benefit residents. This managerial response has focused primarily on preventing infections or direct injuries and the strategies for doing so tend to be top-down, without taking workers' knowledge into account. In focusing on hazardous incidents, the injurious cumulative conditions of laundry work are often normalized. We more frequently saw managers seeking ways to accommodate such hazards as rushing rather than addressing the overwhelming workloads and insufficient staffing levels that cause this rush. Efforts to address occupational health and safety that focus primarily on discrete points of potential physical harm are too narrow in scope to address harmful working conditions.

Despite the recognition that laundry and clothing work can pose a significant health risk, the failure to provide enough workers, enough resources, and appropriate physical designs to ensure sanitary conditions can undermine efforts to follow infection control strategies and to prevent other risks. Many of these failures are themselves the product of strategies intended to enhance efficiency. In other words, efficiency strategies can lead to increased risks and lower quality of care in the long run.

WORKERS' STRATEGIES FOR RISK MANAGEMENT

When workplace injury prevention policies and managerial strategies do not sufficiently address workers' experiences with hazardous working conditions, they often develop their own strategies for protecting themselves. As argued by Day (2014), workers are not merely passive victims of dangerous working conditions, but rather devise strategies to cope with and mitigate the risk of physical injury, gendered and racialized abuse, and the job-jeopardizing perception that they have done their work insufficiently or incorrectly. By examining these strategies, we can better understand the dangerous conditions that workers face in performing laundry work.

The most obvious collective strategy is unionization. Except in the United States, all the workplaces we visited are unionized. Without a union, workers have few ways to resist workplace risks, especially when it is overall working conditions that undermine health. That the

Texas workers we interviewed get only five paid days each year with which to cover vacation and illness speaks volumes about the importance of unions to workplace health. As we discussed in chapter 1, unions have helped mitigate some of the most obvious aspects of precarity such as low wages and lack of benefits and sick leave, which are critical to health. Unions can also provide workers with a voice and prevent unreasonable dismissal. Moreover, unions are usually participants in workplace health and safety committees where policies are developed and where workers can help ensure safety measures are enforced.

Collective bargaining in some instances supported frequent job rotation as a means of reducing injury. Unions in Scandinavia and Canada have also negotiated return-to-work strategies. In a Norwegian home, a combination of union, managerial, and government-led initiatives have resulted in special funding for workers returning to work after illness or injury, as this administrator explained (as translated during the interview by our interviewer):

ADMINISTRATOR: So actually, they might support special measures you make in order to get them back to working life. You call this, you have a name for such a project supported by such means. You call it shoulder to shoulder ... Standing together, right. And ... you try as far as possible to give kind of lighter work at the outset. But ... care work in [a] nursing home is heavy work also physically, so that means that it's a real challenge to try to find the lighter work and it means a lot of considerate planning ...

This extra money, this extra funding for people struggling their way back into working life, they shouldn't be counted as part of the regular staff. They should be in addition to the regular staff because they have extra funding.

INTERVIEWER: That helps the pressure on the other workers.

ADMINISTRATOR: Sure. So it should make them much more positive.

Not surprisingly, it is hard for workers to return to heavy workloads, and not surprisingly other workers resent it if a worker is assigned a lighter load, given the added pressures on them. The strategy of gradual return that does not count on regular staffing shouldering the extra burden addressed these problems, offering an example of how structural approaches can work. In other words, collective strategies that involve workers are required, and these strategies need to take structural factors into account.

In one Canadian home, the workers were successful in their demands for air conditioning, but unions have been less successful in resisting privatization and other managerial strategies identified above that can undermine health. In our interviews with local union representatives, we heard about the frustration of being told cutbacks meant nothing could be done. And from workers, we heard frustration with unions' waning power and inability to resist. One example of union failure was a managerial policy to require colour-coded polyester uniforms. Workers found the uniforms uncomfortable and inappropriate for their work, making their work more difficult. Although the union objected, it failed to change this management decision. Nevertheless, workers do use their unions to address some risks, prompting on occasion changes that have a wider impact. In Manitoba, for example, the union worked with the manager to ensure regular part-time work that meant greater safety for residents and staff as a result of the familiarity with the workplace and the residents.

Workers also develop less formal strategies. Although most of these strategies are quite individual, we observed one strategy that did alter the work for everyone. With input from workers and in response to injuries, one workplace put heavy loads of laundry on wheeled carts, thus avoiding the need to lift and carry the load. A more common strategy of workers we interviewed was to obtain a doctor's note, not only to legitimize the workers' injuries but also to prescribe modifications that can accommodate their injuries. One example was prescribed limits on the volume of laundry a worker could be required to push. That these modifications are made through appeal to and the intervention of medical authority speaks not only to the difficulties that workers face in having their injuries recognized in connection to the workplace, but also to their lower position on the hierarchy of care work.

Workers also try to change jobs as a means of escaping the risks of laundry work, often with the help of a union. One laundry worker in a Norwegian nursing home suffered such terrible pain that her doctor wrote a letter to the management recommending she be retrained as a care assistant instead. She explained that care work would actually "be better for my health" and not simply a matter of prevention. This is particularly striking considering the numerous documented hazards associated with care work, including violence, stress, and exhaustion (Armstrong et al. 2011; Armstrong et al. 2009; Banerjee et al. 2008; Banerjee 2010; Daly et al. 2011). For this worker, these risks were actually preferable to the pain she experienced in her laundry job.

When the strains and pains of laundry work are not recognized, often the onus is on workers themselves to manage the risks associated with the laundry. Consider, for example, the preparation regimen of a cleaner at an Ontario nursing home facing eventual rotation into laundry room duties: "I have a year to get ready for it. I talked to my doctor and I have a year to get ready for it. She says, 'Get your core as strong as you can. Walk as much as you can. Get everything as strong as you can. Lift a little bit of weights as much as you can ...' I know how to shortcut to protect my back. She says, 'Do whatever you can to protect yourself and if you injure yourself after you've done all that, then [management] deserves what happens.'" She did whatever she could to strengthen her body in resistance to injurious working conditions, but she did it on her own time and her own initiative. Furthermore, such preparations are necessary in order to make a good case for compensation and/or accommodation should she become injured on the job. Her experiences speak to the challenges these workers face in having hazardous working conditions recognized and counted as such.

A somewhat more collective response is to share the work, using a team approach to mitigate potential harms. We saw many examples of workers informally working in teams to strip beds and sort laundry, demonstrating how workers may collectively strategize to "make it work" amidst overwhelming workloads (Day 2014). We also saw examples of assistive personnel organizing their work so they could together dress or undress a resident who was physically difficult to dress or was agitated and thus more likely to strike out at the worker. We were told of their switching assignments to avoid residents who made racist comments or who became agitated when a man came to provide care. Even workers who have little formal input in care planning processes retain some decision-making capacity to shape their daily work experiences, including decisions about how to protect themselves from various harms.

In sum, workers are active individually and collectively in shaping the health and mitigating the hazards of their workplace environments. This activity, however, is especially limited for those without a union, and workers reported to us that even with a union it is getting harder to protect their health.

CONCLUSION:
THE CONDITIONS OF WORK ARE THE CONDITIONS OF CARE

Laundry and clothes play a significant role in maintaining a healthy and sanitary nursing home environment. However, while laundry workers are positioned as the "guardians of safety" (Andrews 2013) in implementing infection control strategies, the effectiveness of these strategies can be compromised when the conditions of work are neglected. Furthermore, strategies to enhance "efficiency" such as staffing cuts, downsizing, and outsourcing can all impact workers' ability to maintain healthy environments. Although these same working conditions shape the numerous occupational health and safety risks workers face, these risks tend to be poorly recognized and are too often addressed in ways that fail to account for workers' experiences.

Governments, unions, and managers all develop some strategies to address health hazards. And some of those strategies – such as requiring health and safety committees that include workers, providing gloves and the opportunity to wear them, creating pleasant, accessible laundry rooms, and negotiating secure employment – can promote healthy environments. But much more needs to be done to reduce the high illness and injury rates in nursing homes and to make the environments safe for residents without compromising their care.

As the conditions of work are also the conditions of care, there are consequences for residents in failing to recognize occupational risks. If laundry workers are ill, injured, undervalued, and/or excluded from the care team, it is more difficult to provide continuity in care or to develop the care relationship. If laundry and clothing work is not understood as a potential hazard, it is more difficult to provide safe care. Ignoring the risks to workers or treating them in ways that do not address the underlying conditions also has long-term costs in turnover, sick leave, and workers' compensation for the nursing home itself (OECD 2011). Collectively this evidence suggests that addressing laundry workers' injurious working conditions is not merely a matter of boosting staffing levels and morale, nor of changing how the work is organized (Campbell 2013). Rather, we are challenged to ask different kinds of questions about occupational health and safety, including about how this work and its workers are valued, how the work is divided, how the risks of this work are defined and perceived, and ultimately how these risky working conditions impact care.

4

Clothing, Laundry, and Taking Care

We speak of taking care with how we dress: of taking care of our clothes to ensure they are clean as well as repaired, and of taking care to look nice as indicators of self-respect outside nursing homes. Taking care within nursing homes means paying attention to how clothes support the individual and to the work involved in taking care. In the preceding chapters, we used laundry and clothing to explore the inequitable costs, problematic work organization, and risks to residents, families, and workers that are associated with privatization, narrow definitions of care, and a division of labour that too often understands the work of laundry and clothing as ancillary to medical care, except from an infection-control perspective. We also described the clothing and laundry work, identifying who does what in the complicated choreography of nursing home care. In this chapter, we focus more on the contributions that laundry and clothing work make to what residents, relatives, and workers define as good-quality nursing home care.

We begin by examining the role of clothing and laundry in how residents and workers define good care. Clothing is central to maintaining appearances, to preserving residents' dignity not only by making sure that they are dressed and clean but also by ensuring that the clothing reflects the person. Second, we place clothing within the social environment of nursing homes, exploring how clothes and laundry provide an opportunity to foster relations among residents and with workers and families. We then examine how clothing offers an opportunity for "person-centred" or individualized care. Supporting individuals' clothing preferences is an important means for supporting self-expression and individual identity. At the same time, clothes demonstrate to others that workers are indeed taking care of residents. Such care may be limited, however, by the nursing home setting, by working conditions, and by the contradictory pressures on both residents and workers.

Clothes must be cleaned and kept repaired or replaced. But the issue is larger than avoiding shrinkage, stains, or rips and sewing buttons back on. The state of clothes and how residents are dressed are clear indicators to residents, families, visitors, and other workers of taking care and of respecting individual choices. At the same time, lost or damaged clothing can be a source of conflict between nursing home staff, residents, and their relatives, undermining the care relationship. Residents' involvement in laundry and clothing work can not only provide stimulation but also allow residents the dignity of exercising their skills and choices, offering another indicator of taking care. Similarly, supports that allow residents to dress themselves can contribute to active, healthy aging. All this takes time as well as other resources, and requires some autonomy as well as teamwork among those assigned to provide this care.

DEFINING GOOD CARE:
CLEANLINESS, COMFORT, AND KEEPING UP APPEARANCES

Making sure that residents are "clean and comfortable" was frequently noted by care workers in response to our question "what is good care?" It is a modest ambition but one that must be understood in the context of the various pressures that workers face. For care workers assisting residents with bathing, feeding, toileting, dressing, and the general necessities of daily life, making sure that residents are "clean and comfortable" can be a real challenge – particularly if residents are frail, incontinent, or cognitively impaired, or have limited mobility. Furthermore, when there is insufficient funding, inadequate staffing levels, and problematic work organization, making sure that residents are "clean and comfortable" often represents the most that care workers can accomplish amidst these working conditions.

Yet workers frequently struggle to go beyond this minimum, to extend what "clean and comfortable" means. This was expressed by one frontline care worker at an Ontario nursing home when asked what he thought was good about his job: "After you wash a patient and you know he [feels] good and he's all dressed nice, nice looking, I am happy for him or her. He must feel good or she must feel good. Sometime after we're going to ask, 'Oh, this is still good, eh?' And the patient will say, 'Yes.' Just that. I did my job, you know. Yeah, because it's not too much I could do except giving care, respect the patient." Assistive personnel cannot alter residents' medication, and in many jurisdictions they have little say in the care plan. At the same time, heavy workloads often mean they cannot spend much time talking with the resident, providing them with company, or taking them for an outing. Making sure that residents are "dressed nice" and "feel good" is thus central to care workers' definition of what makes for good care. It can be one of the most important elements when care workers experience a strict division of labour and have limited decision-making capacity in other aspects of care. As there is "not too much" they can do otherwise to shape care, workers can have some control over attending to residents' appearances when time allows. Attending to appearance helps assure workers that they have done the job of care the best they can.

Dress is about more than being comfortable physically. It is also about being comfortable within a given social context. As Entwistle (2001, 48) observes, clothing and appearance are "a way that we demonstrate our participation in the standards of social interaction. Dressed inappropriately for a situation we feel vulnerable and embarrassed and so too when our dress 'fails' us, when in public we find we've lost a button, stained our clothes or find our flies undone." Conversely, being well-dressed according to our personal definitions can give us both pleasure and confidence while reinforcing our individual identity. Moreover, how we are dressed is important to our ability to successfully uphold the standards and expectations of a particular social order. Clothing plays a central role in constituting social difference, and how we are dressed indicates our participation in cultural, class, and gender norms (Twigg 2010). For instance, wearing a bra or fly-fronted pants can be important to a person's embodied gender identity in helping to maintain the performance of normative femininity/masculinity (Twigg 2010). Indeed, dress is one of the primary ways by which gender is performed (Butler 1990). In this sense, taking care is about maintaining residents' dignity through dress that is socially comfortable for residents as well. Comfort is socially defined, and thus is about more than fit or fabric, for "how you are socially presented, with the embedded meanings implied, can be a source of ease and calm – or its reverse" (Twigg 2010, 226). While nursing homes provide a particular social context, the extent to which dress differs from the world outside can indicate the extent to which that world and the identities associated with that world are lost.

We heard from families, workers, and residents about the importance of being dressed appropriately according to social standards of the world outside. As one resident explained, care workers' help with clothing and getting dressed is a part of making sure that a resident is "put together" before leaving their room in the morning. Successfully participating in the performance of acceptable appearance – that is, managing to look "put together" according to norms of culture, class, and gender – is also an important source of pleasure for residents. Consider the conversation one of our researchers had with a resident who was pleased to be dressed in a well-matching outfit:

> I commented on her being a well-dressed woman – the lovely purple blouse and skirt on Tuesday and the red, blue and white blouse combined with a navy skirt today. She told us that she was happy when she found this blouse this morning because she had considered wearing a pink or a white blouse. But that wouldn't have been as smart. We found it amazing how much she is concerned about appearance. And I also think that the physical appearance of residents is evidence of good care work. Staff want their residents to appear in a dignified way in social settings.

The resident's concern over her appearance presents a challenge to assumptions about clothing, gender, and the aging body. We found it "amazing" that the resident was concerned with her appearance, given the assumptions prevalent in many nursing homes about what is possible in this context and deeper assumptions about the elderly and their concern for appearances – especially assumptions about elderly women's appearances. As Twigg (2007) notes, concern over fashion and style tends to be associated with the consumer culture of youth, hence the frequent assumption that an older woman would have less interest in looking smart. Older women's clothing choices and interest in appearance are often neglected based on "assumptions that fashion is all about sexuality and that older people – certainly in the eyes of the young – are beyond sex" (Twigg 2007, 287). This assumption may be even more commonly made about those who live in nursing homes, where most residents are significantly challenged both physically and cognitively.

However, being well-dressed is an important part of older persons' strategies for maintaining dignity, as clothing is a part not only of our gendered performance, but also of our outward presentation of social status and mental capacity. Clothing that is dirty, damaged, or otherwise socially inappropriate is damaging to self-respect (Calnan, Badcott, and Woolhead 2006). It invokes the image of the decrepit "dementia patient" and the associated incapacity of frail old age (Twigg 2010, 228). Attention to maintaining a socially acceptable appearance persists even among residents with severe cognitive and physical decline (Kontos 2004) – conditions that are challenging to one's dignity. Being dressed smartly may thus be one of the few ways that residents can maintain a sense of dignity amidst otherwise undignified circumstances, and can help residents in "subverting expectations of what a frail older person would look like" (Buse and Twigg 2015, 14).

In nursing home settings, where residents often depend on care workers for some or total assistance in getting dressed, making sure that residents are dressed with dignity is not only about the end result of appearances, but also about the social processes involved in being dressed by others. For example, at a Nova Scotia home that followed a model with an explicit policy of person-centred care, we observed two care workers having a thoughtful discussion about whether a resident was appropriately dressed. She wore a green sweater with a blue blouse: one care worker was concerned that these colours clashed, while the other thought the colours worked well together. The resident was not an object of the discussion, but rather was fully included as a participant in the conversation despite having great difficulty with speaking. Maintaining a dignified appearance in residential care is thus not just about what residents are wearing, but also about whether and how residents are involved in the process. This encounter also speaks to care workers' role in maintaining "some semblance of gendered normality" (Lee-Treweek 1997, 53) in the process of dressing residents. Concern over dress is culturally constituted as a feminine activity (Twigg 2007), and in this sense a discussion around whether the resident's clothing did or did not clash constitutes the performance of a particularly gendered script in relation to clothing and appearance.

While we saw plenty of examples of workers taking care to ensure residents were dressed in ways that reflected their individual identities and respected their dignity, we also saw instances of the reverse. In a UK home, for example, we saw men walking around with soiled and smelly pants. This small, privately owned home in an old house had many rooms that may have made it difficult for staff to keep track of residents. Space issues were compounded by limited staffing levels. Staff were rushing around on narrow stairs with a gate at the bottom that they had to manually open each time they went up or down. Low staffing levels were also a factor in Canada where we witnessed residents with food from breakfast stuck to the front of their clothing as they watched TV. These instances stood out to us in our field notes as moments when residents' appearances clearly did not fit with acceptable norms, creating a stark differentiation between these residents and those we noted as being "smart" or well-dressed – illustrating that it is not just what one wears, but also the cleanliness of one's clothing that plays a role in creating and maintaining social difference.

Incorporating attention to dress into the definition of respectful care may be as important for the relatives of nursing home residents as it is for residents themselves. Clean, neat and orderly, and even fashionable appearances often serve as a barometer of good care and residents' well-being (Ward et al. 2008, 640). As one Swedish care worker put it, making sure that "Mom and Dad [look] to have it good – clean and nice" is a part of how care workers manage relatives' expectations for good nursing home care. Family members are not around for the majority of body work involved in nursing home care, work that takes place behind the closed doors of residents' rooms and bathrooms. A resident's appearance, however, provides a visible and daily indicator of taking care. Seeing residents dressed appropriately may assure family members that their relative is being treated well – a particular concern amidst increased emphasis on accountability in long-term care regulation. A care worker at a Texas nursing home drew on familial imagery to explain the importance of making sure that residents "look presentable," as this is how she would like her own relative to be treated: "Mostly I'm just feeding them or making sure their clothes are nice and clean. I try to make sure they look presentable because if their family comes in I would want my grandma to look like she was taken care of. I wouldn't want her to be like sitting in a corner over there like slouched down, you know. So I basically think of it as how would I want my grandma treated is how I treat them." For this care worker, making sure that residents are dressed well helps to reassure family members that residents are being well cared for, a clear indicator that attention has been paid to the resident, that Mom or Dad has not been forgotten and left "slouched down in a corner." Making sure that residents are "presentable" for their family members may thus help care workers to manage relatives' fears about residential care as inferior to home-based care, given the idealization of the family and home as a source of loving, respectful, and best-quality care. Conversely, we heard from many workers that families often complain about how the resident is dressed, creating tension and sometimes reprimands for the workers.

But workers still make the effort even when there are no relatives to monitor the care through clothes. A staff member at a US nursing home explained that investing in residents' appearances is important whatever the circumstances of the resident: "You got to look at the residents making sure that they're clean. You know, they don't have raggedy clothes on. You know, you have money in your budget that you have to look at okay, this person doesn't have any family, okay. But they look raggedy. You've got to buy them some clothes. You've got to get them a haircut and things like that."

In sum, although workers often report that good care is defined by keeping residents clean and comfortable and although conditions often make it difficult to do more than this, we saw plenty of evidence of workers going beyond this minimum. The relatives expect more, and good grooming is an obvious visible measure for them of respectful care. But workers make the effort to make residents "look nice" even in the absence of relatives, taking care in ways that give workers the satisfaction of seeing the pleasure and comfort it brings.

CLOTHES AND THE SOCIAL ENVIRONMENT

Clothing also has an impact on the social environment, offering opportunities in nursing homes to foster social interaction among residents, between residents and staff, and with families and volunteers (Charras and Gzil 2013). Yet the social environment tends to be neglected amidst medicalized and market-driven approaches to nursing home care.

Clothing invites conversation. Like others (Powers 2003), we noticed that residents comment on and talk with one another about clothing. For instance, we observed two women residents complimenting each other warmly on their clothing over lunch, telling one another "you look very smart" and "your dress is very pretty too." Attending to each other's clothing was a way of continuing to act out a particularly gendered script between these two women, given the association of concern over appearance with normative femininity. Workers too use clothing as a means of starting conversations and similarly maintaining gendered norms, commenting on how nice residents look to the delight of residents and workers alike. When they have time to "dress up" residents, as we observed during Christmas celebrations in a BC home, the importance of clothes both for the dignity of residents and as a basis for social interaction with workers was particularly obvious.

But clothing and appearance are not only important for those residents who are women, nor is it only important to workers to ensure that the women they care for are dressed well. Consider the following observation from our field notes at an Ontario nursing home, where a care worker's efforts at dressing and grooming a male resident fostered social interaction and the playing out of gendered practices among multiple residents and staff:

> Suddenly there is a happy-sounding commotion off to the side hallway, "look who's up and smiling!" One of the care aides wheels a resident out into the hallway wearing his legion hat and all dressed up. She tells me "I just bathed him and did his hair, look how nice he looks!" As she wheels him over in his wheelchair the RPN [registered practical nurse] says to the resident "WOW aren't you sexy!" She holds his hand as he passes by. "Eh

you're looking really sexy today!" The resident smiles but says nothing, the care aide and RPN laugh [kindly, not mockingly]; care aide wheels the resident towards the dining rooms.

As this interaction was happening, another resident was looking on and required assistance with a laundry basket. As the RPN moved to help him, she included him in the efforts of "looking really sexy": "He calls out to the RPN, 'nurse, can you help me?' RPN goes over, 'doing some laundry eh?' lifts the basket onto his lap. She adjusts his shirt for him too, which had ridden up on his stomach when he attempted to reach down for the basket, and she fixes the collar of his sweater jacket. She says to him, 'There, now you look sexy too!' Peter chuckles a bit and drives his chair down the hallway." The care aide dressing the resident in his legion uniform and carefully grooming him for the day invited social interaction between residents and staff, a playful moment that residents appeared to genuinely enjoy. Staff too appeared to be very happy to see the first resident up and nicely groomed despite being, as we would later learn, one of the most physically frail residents at the home, which meant he required total assistance with daily activities. Dressing the resident in his legion uniform also conveys to others something about the resident's biography. Furthermore, in telling the first resident that he was "looking really sexy" and then extending the "sexy" compliment to the other male resident as well, the nurse (a woman) also invoked heterosexual norms to reaffirm the residents' masculinity.

Dressing can also invite other forms of social interaction. Our research team found that clothing was often a way into residents' stories of and memories about their past, illustrating how clothing additionally contributes to the social environment as a storytelling tool (Buse and Twigg 2016). Visitors and volunteers also often used clothing as a starting point to conversation, and as an indicator of how the resident was feeling today. Clothing suggested a personal history or current attitudes that provided a basis for social interaction.

Workers' clothing can also make a difference to the broader social environment, shaping the interactions between residents, relatives, and staff (Charras and Gzil 2013). In some homes staff clothing choices were specifically intended to foster social interaction with residents. For instance, an activity coordinator at an Ontario nursing home wore amusing clothing for residents to comment on during holiday singalongs and social events. Care staff also used costume clothing to prompt conversation among residents, as in the case of one UK home we visited. At this home, wearing brightly coloured clothing, jewellery, and other accessories such as boas and big flowers is explicitly a part of the home's approach to care. Staff are encouraged to vary their clothing as a means of drawing residents' attention, particularly residents with dementia. The manager of this home explained to us how important it was to avoid uniforms and to allow workers the freedom to wear clothing creatively, citing that uniforms create undesirable "barriers" of inequality between staff and residents. A family member of a resident at this home explained what a difference this makes in how staff and residents relate to one another, comparing the home's no-uniform policy with the more "medical" look of homes where uniforms are used:

> I think that helps to reassure the residents … because the white, the outfits that other people have worn I think imply a medical authority in some way, and I think that's unsettling when they don't know where they are and they don't know what's happening and why are all these people around in white coats, you know. It's not ideal. So I much prefer that. I've heard some people, not here but the view that would take away sort of the element of professionalism … I think that's another issue you've got to be aware of, but as long as that is preserved – and I've not seen anything to suggest it wouldn't be – I think that's better for what they're trying to do with the place and sort of go with the flow and, you know, all that. Well, that's not how [it is] if you've got people in white coats saying "Don't do that" all the time. They did have those in the other place Dad was at. It just felt wrong, really.

As this relative notes, uniforms imply not only a certain type of authority, but also a particular type of social interaction associated with that authority: a proscriptive, surveillance-like approach, wherein residents are monitored and medically managed. In contrast, this relative felt that workers' lack of uniforms at this home reflected their go-with-the-flow approach to interacting with residents. Similarly, a volunteer at this same home appreciated how the removal of uniforms helped to make everyone "more approachable for visitors."

The role of clothing in fostering social interaction and cultivating the relationship between staff and residents was quite keenly expressed in one Ontario nursing home where uniforms had recently been implemented for most staff. The director, an RN, justified the introduction of uniforms in two ways. First, uniforms would allow residents and visitors to distinguish more easily among types of care workers, differentiating assistive personnel from registered care workers from cleaners, etc. And second, uniforms would help eliminate sanitation risks in the case of workers who were wearing the same clothes to multiple job sites – a common occurrence given the low wages and lack of full-time employment in nursing homes. However, in addition to the personal costs incurred from having to purchase new clothes, staff found that a significant downside to this change is that they have lost a crucial conversation topic with residents. One care worker explained what a loss this was for staff and residents alike:

CARE WORKER: The colours and the patterns, they [the residents] used to love that. But now it's just one colour so it's like if they see this colour every day it's like come on, you know.
INTERVIEWER: How long have you had this colour?
CARE WORKER: Just since a couple months now. Since December. They changed us into this one colour.
INTERVIEWER: I saw the photograph in the photo gallery.
CARE WORKER: Yeah, we used to have …
INTERVIEWER: A splendid array of colours, flowers.
CARE WORKER: Yeah, we used to have that down there and they used to love that, you know, but they just put us in one colour now so it's like oh blah. We used to wear a lot of different pattern[s] and stuff and we used to get a lot of compliment[s] and they'll come and touch it. "Oh, a cat" or "That's a moon," you know. We find them more active like that. But just this one colour they see every day is dull.
INTERVIEWER: It's a beautiful colour.
CARE WORKER: It is but not the colour that we used to wear and the different patterns. Now. Especially the shirt. Different colours

and different pattern[s] for them. They like bright colour. They like the patterns and the colour. They'll come and say, "Oh, that's a cat." "Oh, that's a dog." And I have one with the moon and stars. I always have this lady come up. "Oh, I like your top. It's beautiful. That's a moon. That's ..." You know? Then they get, actually, their mind is off. They get distracted and then you can get along with them more. But with this one colour ...

INTERVIEWER: For you as workers is it better to have the same colour? Does it help you at all? You're shaking your head.

CARE WORKER: No.

INTERVIEWER: It's no different.

CARE WORKER: No. It was just a nurse scrub in a uniform, you know. You could wear a different uniform every day but [now] get up every day and one uniform. You don't change your uniform today. You know? Just one. Everybody is in green and black. Black and green.

Previously workers at this nursing home wore brightly coloured scrubs of their own choice, which resulted in many different patterns on their shirts. The colours, they told us, helped divert residents' attention and made it so that workers could "get along" better with them. Residents appreciated and would comment on workers' clothing. This was quite important in particular for the assistive personnel who perform the majority of hands-on bodily care. Another care worker noted that what she wears is not just utilitarian, but rather an expression of a "state of heart" in relating to residents. She took pride in cultivating an extensive work wardrobe of different patterned scrubs for residents to enjoy. Now, however, she explained that it is "like we're in a prison" with everyone in the same colour. Workers have not only lost a crucial conversation starter with residents, they have also lost a source of pleasure and pride in their work. And they have lost a process that promotes relational care. The union was unsuccessful in resisting the change, in part, we were told, because there was a trade-off with the compensation for the uniforms.

A PERSON-CENTRED APPROACH:
IDENTITY, PREFERENCES, AND CHOICE

As Twigg (2010) argues, clothing is intimately tied to our sense of self. Our clothing practices are tied to gender, class, and culture and are reflective of our individual tastes and preferences. Clothing is thus a part of one's "embodied identity" (Buse and Twigg 2015). The expression of identity through clothing may be a particularly important issue for persons residing in nursing homes, where individuals' identities are challenged by routines, rules, and declining physical health and cognition. In this sense, personal clothing holds important significance for residents as a source of expression of selfhood amidst the potentially depersonalizing and institutionalizing processes of nursing home care.

The important role of clothing in residents' expressions of cultural, class, and gender identity was clear in all our observations. For instance, at an Ontario nursing home we observed a resident wearing a beaded necklace and earrings that suggested her Indigenous identity. At an expensive private nursing home in Texas where it was possible to have clothes sent out for cleaning, our field notes recorded residents wearing costly fabrics like silk. And observations from a Norwegian nursing home illustrate very clearly the role that clothing plays in maintaining residents' feminine and masculine identities:

Many of the ladies I see are wearing a cardigan over a nice blouse, with either a long skirt (as the frowning lady wears) or matching slacks. The lady with the dangling earrings also wears a matching necklace and a beaded headband, her hair nicely arranged around the headband and I think that she is wearing some lip colour. Lillian's hair has been curled and is neatly arranged. Hans has been nicely dressed in trousers and a wool sweater. I think that staff must put a lot of effort into getting residents dressed and groomed for the day – even for Hans, the least mobile of the group, who could easily have been in pjs all day but isn't. Even the "smiling lady" who I saw sitting in [the] kitchen, who is dressed more casually in a sweater and pants, had been wearing matching colours (pink sweater with pink pants).

Makeup, accessories, and matching clothing all assist the women in this scene with maintaining the gendered expectation of women's attention to appearances, while the completely immobile and dependent Hans is dressed in gender-appropriate trousers even though they may be difficult to put on when he is in a wheelchair. The high staffing levels, combined with the importance attached to care for older people, supported this approach.

In our study, the link between clothing and identity often arose around the central theme of choice, with either residents themselves or their care providers saying that adhering to individuals' clothing preferences and choices is an important element in taking care. Choosing one's own clothing has been found to be important to residents' self-esteem in institutional settings, enhancing residents' quality of life by offering an opportunity for control and autonomy in institutional settings (Chowdhary 1991). Given the link between clothing and identity, asserting one's clothing preferences in nursing home care may also be a way of carving out space for individual expression amidst the depersonalizing routines of nursing home life (Harnett 2010).

We found that incorporating clothing preferences into nursing homes' approach to care took two different forms: first, as a continuation of a resident's lifelong preferences for a particular style of dress, and second as an ongoing conversation about or negotiation of clothing choice. As an example of the former approach, a friend of one resident at a German nursing home noted the importance of being dressed in clothing that reflected the resident's established preferences for matching clothing: "After they've had their meals the nurses take care, make sure that their hands are washed and cleaned. And for [the resident] it's very important that everything she wears the colours are speaking to each other, not just anything but it all matches. From the very beginning she had the opportunity to set up preferences, the way she'd like everything done like with the hairdresser, going to getting a pedicure done, all those things she was able to discuss with the nurses and set it up according to the way she would like it done. It's all done according to the way she wants it." For this resident, being dressed in matching colours, and not "just anything," such as mismatched or hastily chosen clothing, is an important part of good care because it means she is able to have her previously expressed preferences carried out by care staff. These personal preferences were set up upon entering the care home and formed a part of her individual care plan. The care plan structure, supported by adequate staffing levels and the value attached to older people, helped make clothing a priority.

At a Manitoba nursing home, a manager explained to us that recording resident clothing preferences in this manner was an example of the most important information in the resident care plan for care workers, and a part of what made her nursing home unique:

> Our care plans are not always the same as other peoples' and they're much more identifiable and individual. So if the care plan says this lady likes wearing a pink sock and a green sock that's what we care plan. We don't take that sort of picked one that says, you know, [the] resident will wear socks because invariably [the] resident is not going to wear the same pair. So because the care plan has to be something that if you take it you can go off and give care. You know, it will say, "This lady will not wear a sweater" or "Do not use a brush on her hair." So it sort of gives all of that information because that's the valuable part of the care plan.

Reflecting the link between clothing and respectful care, using the care plan to take care in this home involves attention to residents' individual preferences for clothing and grooming. This manager was able to create a unique care plan in part because she created the policy for this new home and in part because the government gave her considerable autonomy when she was setting up the home.

The loss of ability to express one's identity and established clothing preferences may be particularly difficult for residents suffering from dementia (Twigg and Buse 2013), representing an additional layer of loss atop the already difficult transition to a nursing home. For example, a relative of a resident at an Ontario nursing home told us that her family member, who now has Alzheimer's, would be "devastated" if he knew that he was not being dressed neatly, as he always preferred a neat and stylish appearance in his life prior to being in a nursing home. Although Ontario nursing homes are highly regulated, the priority in the mandated care plans is physical indicators of care, and we saw little evidence that the non-physical data collected are given high priority when care plans are translated into action.

Clothing choice can also be approached as an ongoing, negotiated process in the daily work of care, as a way of personalizing the care process. For instance, one east coast home in our study that follows an explicit person-centred model has made resident clothing choice an explicit part of its person-centred model of care, with workers asking residents their clothing preferences as they get them up and dressed for the day. This approach was reflected in the diversity of dress and appearance among residents, as we observed in our field notes: "Accessories and styles of dress are just one way in which you can see that this is quite personalized. Some residents are dressed up, with scarves and jewelry, and others are very much more casual in their dress. Some women wear trousers and others wear skirts and blouses."

At a Swedish nursing home, a care worker told us that residents choose what they wear on a day-to-day basis, whether that was their everyday clothes or a bathrobe that day. As she explained, what residents wear "depends on what they want," and it is the job of care workers to respect that choice. Other nursing homes seemed to support resident clothing choices in practice even when these choices might conflict with safety concerns or clothing norms, as evidenced by residents wearing heeled footwear despite using a walker or wearing multiple layers of blouses without having this unconventional clothing choice corrected by care workers. As one family member at a UK nursing home noted, allowing residents to make these daily choices about their own clothing, rather than dressing residents in what she called a "uniform of ease" (that is, in whatever is easiest for care workers to locate, put on, and take off), is a way of preserving residents' dignity. The practice was supported by the model followed by the nursing home.

It is important to note that care workers are not alone in the role of supporting residents' daily clothing choices. For instance, at one UK nursing home where laundry is processed on site, laundry workers were well acquainted with the preferences of residents, knowing for example that one resident in particular liked his shirts to be crisply ironed because "he's a man that likes smart clothes." Laundry workers may also be able to support residents' clothing preferences through the types of equipment that they have, such as machines that allow them to wash delicate clothing or woollen items. These examples speak of the potential for laundry workers to support resident preferences, given sufficient equipment as well as being sufficiently incorporated into the care team to be able to develop knowledge about individual residents' clothing preferences.

However, there are some challenges and limitations to supporting residents' identities and preferences through clothing, exemplifying limitations to the idealized notion of personalized or person-centred care. The nursing home environment and the processes of care can limit residents' clothing choices, beginning with the resident's admission to the home. The handbook given to new residents and their relatives upon moving into one Canadian nursing home recommends that resident clothing be washable and dryable, in at least a seven-day supply, and "comfortable and easy to put on and take off"; that is, easy for care workers to manage in the processes of bodily care. Interestingly, the *Resident Bill of Rights* (required by government regulations) in this home also states that residents have the right to "clothing of their own choice." But the handbook guidelines clearly show that this choice is restricted by the possibilities of this home's laundry and care processes. The warning that clothes should be "washable and dryable" impacts the kinds of clothing that residents can have in terms of material and texture. Delicates and natural fibres such as silk or wool can be easily destroyed in commercial machines, requiring special equipment and sufficient staff time to separate and appropriately wash these materials. Only a few homes in our study with in-house laundry had the capacity to handle such materials, while homes that outsource their laundry could not do so at all. Not only does this make a difference for residents' ability to maintain their preferred style of dress, it also makes a difference for residents' experience of wearing clothing and being comfortable.

In another home's collection of resident guidelines, residents are also advised how much of each item of clothing to bring, reminiscent of summer camp packing lists – the number of socks, pants, etc. to supply. Residents and/or their relatives assisting with their admission are advised in the orientation guide of yet another home that the clothing one brings to the facility "should reflect the resident's current lifestyle" – noting that "numerous" dresses and sweaters are "not needed" in the nursing home setting, and that there is limited space in residents' rooms for storing clothing. Choice, then, is restricted by the fact that residents' personal space in a nursing home is limited to their rooms – especially in shared rooms. Furthermore, the "current lifestyle" implied in the nursing home clothing guidelines is one of practicality, minimalism, and detachment from personal possessions, suggesting residents have reached a point in their lives where having an abundance of clothing choices is no longer necessary. As Twigg (2010, 227) has observed, this process of whittling down residents' wardrobes can be seen as "symbolic as well as practical, marking the deeper transition in to a status on the margins" as personal possessions and their associated status, meanings, and memories are given up, given away, or lost in the transition to nursing home life. It is also reflective of an assumption that nursing home residents experience a diminished role in public life, as "dressing up" clothing and outdoor clothing are pared from residents' wardrobes (Buse and Twigg 2014).

This was not the case everywhere, though, and in some homes we saw possibilities for alternatives. In Sweden, where the residents in the homes we visited had rooms more like bachelor apartments, there was more space for clothes. Near the door in one such apartment was a bench and hooks for outside clothes. The bench was to sit on while putting on boots while the outdoor clothes on the hooks indicate the possibility of leaving, more closely resembling a homelike environment and supporting ongoing engagement in public life.

Space, ideas, and regulations are not the only limits on clothing, though. Not all resident clothing preferences are ideal from the perspective of safety or the practicalities of care provision. Allowing residents to choose their clothing may cause issues for monitoring and maintaining cleanliness. In our field notes at one Ontario home, we observed that while some residents appeared to be able to dress themselves and choose their own clothing, it was unclear whether these residents were being sufficiently monitored by care workers to make sure that their clothing was being regularly changed and laundered, as some wore the same clothing repeatedly. In a Texas home, one resident wore exactly the same beige clothes every day, prompting us to ask in our notes if she simply had clothes that were all the same or if her clothes were not being changed.

There is also the dilemma of how to negotiate between residents' previously expressed preferences and changes to these preferences over time, representing a disruption in the continuity of identity (Buse and Twigg 2015). For instance, the granddaughter of a resident at an Ontario nursing home explained to us that her grandmother had previously always liked to dress up nicely, and to wear fine clothes, as "she has a strong feeling for quality. But during recent months, her interest in jewellery and clothing has decreased." How should care workers respond to this change in interests: by honouring the resident's previous preference for dressing, or by respecting her apparent current lack of interest? Preferences, tastes, and interests can change, and for care workers faced with the job of dressing residents, it is not always clear what constitutes a respectful approach. Furthermore, getting it wrong in dressing a resident can have serious consequences for care workers, including violent outbursts from residents during the dressing process or backlash from upset family members who disapprove of how the resident is dressed.

Workers' ability to support residents' clothing preferences is also limited by how much time they have to perform personal care. As noted above, care plans may contain details about residents' preferences for clothing, which is valuable for supporting a person-centred approach to care. However, care plans are quite lengthy documents and, as one manager noted, "who has time to go through that every day" to make sure that resident clothing preferences are being observed? To address this concern, the Manitoban facility in our study that is led by an innovative manager who got to set up a new home implemented a simplified one-sheet system for residents' clothing and other preferences. Taped inside the door of the resident's closet for easier access, it was a sort of cheat sheet for care workers that they could quickly check when dressing residents.

However, we heard that workers can face challenges in having time constraints recognized by management, who may interpret failure to support residents' clothing choices as a failure of individual staff, a lack of training, or a product of workplace culture rather than a symptom of too little time and burdensome workloads:

MANAGER: Even if it's two choices, right? Do you think you should wear the red or the blue today? What do you think? That takes ten seconds. But we don't do it because we're so focused on just getting the job done. And I wouldn't say that's 100 per cent because I do see situations where they've done beautiful hair and they know somebody loves an outfit and they put it on. So I'm not saying it's 100 per cent across the board. What I would like is if 100 per cent of our people who were asked about it who are capable of making those choices are at least offered the opportunity to make the choice. And we [surveyed] like sixty people. Apparently they are not being asked. That's no cost, that's a limited cost. That's just about the care provider stopping, checking. Yeah, I guess that's time but it's not that much time in the big scale of things, not really.

INTERVIEWER: So how would you shift that? It's kind of like a tiny cultural shift.

MANAGER: I think it's just modelling, conversations, coaching.

While this manager clearly recognizes the importance of clothing, her strategy for promoting residents' clothing choices through additional education that provides "modelling and coaching" for care staff does not address workers' struggles with issues such as understaffing, which can affect how much time workers have to engage residents in conversation about their clothes. If residents are not being asked about what clothing they would like to wear, it is important to consider whether care workers have the time to engage with residents, to find out their preferences, and to support their choices accordingly.

Finally, resident clothing preferences do not always mesh with regulatory requirements in some jurisdictions. One facility manager in Ontario explained to us how regulations requiring residents be "up and dressed" can clash with the mandate to provide a person-centred approach to care. On the one hand, she understands the need for regulations, noting, "I think the standards are there for a good reason because I think it elevates good practice in long-term care and, you know, it identifies those homes that require more assistance in order to get there." On the other hand, such rules can conflict with the need for person-centred care. She eloquently identifies the tension:

But at the same [time] it feels very, I don't know, prescriptive in what they tell us we can and can't do and you have to have this and this and this ... You know, we just went through a ministry inspection and upon reading some of their findings ... they were talking about, you know, a resident was found with a purple brief but they're supposed to be in a blue brief and, you know, the staff member was changing the brief and providing good care but they elected to put on a blue one rather than a purple one so that was a finding, you know, and in my heart I'm thinking okay, but the resident was clean and dry and the staff member was providing care so what's the big deal? [laughs] You know, that's my philosophy. And same if a resident wants to sit in their pyjamas all day, why not let them? I do that at home if I'm having a home day and I'm at home and I'm doing laundry and I'm not going anywhere ... I'll shower and put my PJs back on and just, you know, lounge for the day because that's what you do at your home. So it's just very interesting. They want home-like environment. They want you to do all these things in order to personalize the residents' care but at the same time when you really get down to the nitty-gritty, they're very prescriptive and they determine what you can and can't do in long-term care and sometimes you feel constricted.

In some jurisdictions, regulations constrain workers' abilities to respond to resident clothing preferences in a person-centred way, requiring residents to be up and dressed at a particular time. This can cause unnecessary distress for residents and restrict care workers' ability to tailor care to individual resident preferences.

The rules and regulations of the nursing home also make a difference in supporting residents' preferences. Consider the difference that one UK care worker noted when the nursing home she works in transitioned to a person-centred model of care:

CARE WORKER: Before [person-centred care], you are just task focused. I need to do this and that. I need to finish my job. It's more on task. It's not only the person that you look after. It's not [a] feeling-based approach. I need to do this because this is my job, this is my responsibility. And your focus is just tasks. Wash and dress, give them food, and put them to bed, you know. There's no moments before. There's no time for me to enjoy the company of the residents, you know.

INTERVIEWER: And how did you get that time? Did it give you more time, this model?

CARE WORKER: Sometimes let's say if the resident doesn't want to get changed, before now, "You need to get changed. You need to put your clothes on," blah, blah, blah. With the person-centred care if they don't want to get changed, if the resident wants to wear [a] nightie, as long as they're comfortable, as long as they're not wet, it's fine. This is their home. They can do whatever they want to do. If they want to spend a few hours in bed, as long as they're clean and comfortable it's all right. And before now, "You have to get up. Everybody needs to be in the lounge." You know. Now if the resident doesn't want to get dressed, as long as they're clean and comfortable and they're happy, they're not distressed, it's fine.

In switching to a model of care that does not require residents to be dressed in a particular way at a particular time if they do not wish to be, residents are able to make the choice to stay in their pyjamas if they wish. This has also freed care workers from the need to rush to have everyone up and dressed at a specific time, allowing greater flexibility in their day as well as more time for the social care "moments" that this worker describes as being important to respectful care.

Finally, knowledge of resident clothing preferences can make a difference for the quality of care, but this requires a certain type of work organization. An innovative manager at a home in Manitoba explained that part of the home's staffing structure is that all workers have to spend some time with the residents, including the sole in-house laundry worker, who is also responsible for returning clean clothes to residents. As a result, this worker knows her residents very well and is able to tailor the laundry to residents' preferences, at least to the extent that her workload allows, as she explained to us:

INTERVIEWER: Do you get to know the individuals that are on the units, like the residents I mean?

LAUNDRY WORKER: Yeah. Yeah, you do.

INTERVIEWER: So when you're returning their clothes … it's you that does the returning as well?

LAUNDRY WORKER: It is, yeah.

INTERVIEWER: So you get to go in and talk to whoever.

LAUNDRY WORKER: Yeah, and then you kind of know their likes and dislikes and stuff like that.

INTERVIEWER: Can you accommodate that in the laundry, like if they really like this woollen sweater, is that something that you're able to look after in your laundry or not?

LAUNDRY WORKER: I can't do handwashing but say if they wanted it folded a certain way and if I have time to do it then I'll fold their clothes a certain way, or if they want their sweaters in the bottom drawer instead of hung up you kind of get to know that kind of stuff.

Carrying out residents' laundry preferences would be impossible for a worker at an off-site laundry, and would certainly be difficult even for an on-site worker who does not leave the laundry room and is not incorporated into the broader home environment in the same way. Although this worker also noted that while "there's just no time" in her workload to iron residents' clothing or make repairs to clothes that need mending, she can in some smaller ways tailor the laundry care using her knowledge of individuals' preferences.

In sum, given the important role that clothing plays in the expression of individual identity, the ability to choose one's clothing and to have one's clothing preferences supported is an important element in taking care – specifically, taking care in a person-centred way. It is an indicator of autonomy for both the resident and the workers, given that it requires some autonomy in order to put preferences into practice. With some autonomy, there is an opportunity to develop a care relationship. There are, however, limitations to workers' ability to support a person-centred approach to care through clothing. As we discuss further in the next chapter, some of these limitations are very difficult to resolve. However, some of these limitations can be ameliorated by addressing workplace organization, regulations, and the resources available for care, especially if there is support from an understanding manager.

LAUNDRY, LOSS, AND THE CARE RELATIONSHIP

Taking care is not just about ensuring that residents have something clean and comfortable to wear, nor only about making sure that residents can wear clothing of their own choosing. Given the importance of clothing to the care of nursing home residents, taking care also involves ensuring that residents' clothing is undamaged and in good order (Goodwin 1994) – in other words, taking care of residents entails taking care of clothes. As personal possessions, our clothing holds symbolic meaning in being tied to our memories and identities. As a result, the loss of possessions is a challenge to one's personhood and expression of individual will (Powers 2003). It can be particularly upsetting for nursing home residents to have their clothing destroyed or go missing, as this exemplifies the lack of control that residents have over their possessions and environment in institutional life. As one resident put it, noting the indignity of having her clothing mixed up in the laundry, "Why should I see my slacks on another lady?" As we saw, this is a regular occurrence at her nursing home, where personal clothing is collected and washed at a centralized off-site location and often returned to the wrong resident by casual or part-time workers who may not know the residents very well.

In chapter 2, we examined how lost and damaged clothing precipitated the unpaid labour of family members and care workers filling in the gaps when residents' care needs around laundry and clothing are unmet or insufficient. However, an additional issue is the negative impact on the care relationship when things go wrong with the laundry. In our study, problems with lost and damaged clothing were a frequently cited frustration, exemplifying an "iconic" source of conflict in the multi-directional care relationship between residents, relatives, and nursing home staff (Austin et al. 2009, 370). Damaged clothing can be a major frustration for residents – for instance, when clothing is washed at an incorrect temperature so that it no longer fits properly, requiring clothes to be replaced. As observed by others (McGilton et al. 2008), assistive personnel receive the brunt of such complaints, just one of the ways that these care workers must "deal with disappointments" in managing residents' and their relatives' frustrations with unmet expectations of nursing home care. When clothing goes missing, it is care workers who are on the receiving end of family members' outbursts over "where is Mom's this or that," as one care worker in Sweden put it.

Laundry as a source of conflict is not only an issue for care workers. Laundry and cleaning staff are also held accountable for missing or damaged items. At a UK home, laundry workers at the in-house laundry room told us of how "stressed out" residents and family members get when clothing goes missing. One family member was so upset about her relative's missing nighties that she put up pictures of the clothes throughout the nursing home, reminiscent of a "missing person" poster. Another interviewee at a BC nursing home noted that being blamed for missing items was to be expected in working as a cleaner, and that this expectation was explicitly mentioned in her training:

CLEANER: But if it's anything that is missing also that cannot be found ... they will always blame us because we are doing the running around.
INTERVIEWER: Like clothes or something?
CLEANER: Like anything, like maybe jewellery or earrings, anything. And if it cannot be found they will always come to us. And maybe clothes they are blaming us too. We'll never know. But we have to take that because that's what our training guy ... was telling us. "Don't be offended because housekeeping will always get the blame."

As workers who are "doing the running around," housekeeping staff are highly visible and easily accessible staff members as targets of resident/family complaints. Furthermore, as cleaners and laundry workers do not perform hands-on care of residents, relatives may feel safer in complaining about laundry, and thus are more likely to raise this as an issue in their relative's care (Ross, Carswell, and Dalziel 2001).

Avoiding the loss or damage of clothing in the laundry is thus about more than maintaining residents' comfort and appearances, personal choice, or individual expression: it is also about maintaining positive care relationships among residents, relatives, and nursing home staff. The loss or damage of clothing in the laundry can mean lost opportunities for respectful, relational care.

LAUNDRY AS THERAPY AND MEANINGFUL INVOLVEMENT

Being involved in laundry work can serve as a form of therapy for residents with dementia, taking care through meaningful tasks and fostering interaction between staff and residents (Taft et al. 1993). This approach was evident in several of the nursing homes in our study. In these instances, residents were involved in laundry and laundry-related work specifically for the benefits that this activity can have on mood or memory. One worker at a UK nursing home identified resident involvement in laundry as an activity that exemplified why the facility "works," particularly for residents with dementia. She recounts going into a resident's room and "seeing washing" that could be taken up by the resident. The manager "might give her some towels to fold up because then it brings back memories of doing the washing." The activity influences their mood and their behaviour. According to this worker, "nine times out of ten you see them quite relaxed" while they are folding the towels. This resident's memories of doing the laundry transcended her dementia, providing a calming effect through the memory of meaningful household work. Giving her towels to fold is also an example of tailoring the nursing home care to the resident's gendered personal experiences, using knowledge of the resident's biography to make individualized care decisions (Kontos, Miller, and Mitchell 2010).

Laundry is also used to foster active resident involvement in the communal life of the nursing home. As one manager at a Swedish nursing home explained, resident involvement in laundry can be a way of encouraging residents to "focus on the things they could do," a way of fostering residents' independence while contributing to the broader processes of the nursing home. This was less clearly the case at a German nursing home, where residents' folding of napkins and tablecloths is documented as an "occupational activity." Although documented as part of therapeutic programming, some tasks associated with private homes such as loading the dishwasher and helping with meal preparation offered not only meaningful work but also work that was in some instances paid in recognition of the contribution to the work of the home. Similarly, providing residents with clean laundry to fold is one of a variety of "homelike chores" that residents were encouraged to participate in at a BC nursing home in our study, where this chore work was formally integrated into the home's approach to care. Delegating some laundry work to residents offers an opportunity for residents to contribute to the nursing home in a way that is more meaningful, not simply a means of distraction. This approach is also in contrast to a service model or hotel-like approach to nursing home care, wherein resident laundry is provided as a market service for all residents regardless of their individual capacities (Auestad 2010).

However, we found there was a difference between residents' laundry work meaningfully contributing to the activities of the nursing home and it being pointless busywork. Depending on how laundry was included in the "therapeutic milieu" (Taft et al. 1993) of the nursing home environment, it was not always clear whether residents found this activity meaningful. The manager of a Manitoba home told us that residents were given towels to fold "because they have short attention spans," and folding was a task that required minimal focus. Similarly, at an Ontario nursing home, folding towels was used as a way to "keep residents' hands busy." In these instances, folding the laundry appeared to be more of an opportunity to distract residents and occupy their attention, rather than a way to promote meaningful participation in the communal work of residential life.

CONCLUSIONS

Clothing and laundry play central roles in the "taking care" in nursing homes. Maintaining residents' appearances is important to care workers, residents, and their relatives alike, supporting dignified care and assuaging relatives' fears of depersonalized and poor-quality institutional care. What care workers wear also makes a difference for taking care by supporting the social environment. Given the link between clothing and identity, choice of clothing preferences is an important element in person-centred care, and we saw numerous examples of work organization, regulations, care models, and managers who supported the dignity of residents through clothing. However, there are many ways this ideal is often limited in practice by nursing home rules, regulations, and restrictive work organization. Laundry too is important to care, given the conflict that can arise in the care relationship when clothing goes missing, is damaged, or is not kept clean and free of smells. Finally, while laundry can help foster resident involvement in nursing home life, this approach exemplifies the dilemmas that can arise in developing occupational programming for nursing homes around capacity and the gendered assumptions underlying homelike care.

In examining the relationship between clothing, laundry, and care, this analysis has raised broader dilemmas around how to support dignified, respectful, and person-centred care amidst the rules, regulations, competing interests, and workplace organization of a nursing home environment. In the following chapter, we will further explore how laundry and clothing reveal limitations and tensions in the idealized notion of homelike care.

5

Contradictions, Tensions, and Possibilities

Feminist political economy draws our attention not only to economic forces, public policies, structures, and ideas but also to contradictions and tensions that shape practices. There are multiple, contradictory pressures on nursing homes, which create tensions they all face to some degree. These contradictions play out in particular ways in relation to clothes and laundry. In this chapter we reflect back on various themes previously raised and examine them from the perspective of contradictions and tensions, exploring some promising practices used to address or at least balance those pressures in the sites we visited. The overarching contradictions we deal with here are those between home and institution, between autonomy and risk, between communities and individuals, and between short- and long-term strategies. These are not the only contradictions we identified, but they serve to illustrate the complex issues at work and the need to recognize contradictory pressures in struggling to take care.

HOMES AND INSTITUTIONS

At some point in the interviews across all of the nursing homes in all of the countries in our study, staff and/or management talked about these places as homes – or at least expressed the desire for these places to be homelike. What makes a home is of course a matter of debate, and undoubtedly varies with class, gender, and culture (Dyck et al. 2005; Leith 2006). And the meaning of home may also change with age (Frank and Wahl 2000). But Annison's (2000) review of the literature suggests that there is a common agreement that homes should reflect ideas and values, privacy, personal status, and appropriate material conditions, among other factors. As we explained in the previous chapter, the clothes people wear and their condition is one indicator of personal status, a symbol of the extent to which they can control their appearance and maintain their identity as they would at home. Clothes also reflect values, indicating degrees of care and respect. In nursing homes as in private homes, clothes must be cleaned and residents must be dressed. Thus the ways these clothes and laundry are handled have a critical influence on the extent to which long-term care facilities feel and look like anyone's home.

At the same time, these are communal places full of fragile and vulnerable people who often have similar clothes. The focus on the risk of spreading infections not only among residents but also to the people who do the care work that we described in chapter 3 can conflict with efforts to appear homelike and to treat residents in homelike ways. Spending the day in bed or a wheelchair also makes it difficult to wear clothes or dress people in clothes that symbolize the independence of home. These places are at once workplaces and living places, and the demands of the work are different from those in homes, creating another set of tensions. Moreover, in contrast to private homes, state policies have an obvious presence in long-term residential care, and this presence shapes the extent to which these places can be like anyone's home. Although these tensions related to clothes and laundry were visible in all the homes we visited, some managed to balance these tensions in ways that shifted towards a homelike environment.

Laundry and Homes

While it may be difficult to sort out what makes a place homelike for specific populations, laundry can contribute a great deal to whether a place looks like a home or an institution. As our field notes indicate, an Ontario nursing home was anything but homelike:

> The hallway now has a linen trolley and clothes rack outside the bathing room. In the hallway, the PCAs [personal care assistants] are sorting clothes on the racks. The lights in the hall are now turned on and PCAs begin to bring out the empty soiled laundry

bins. There's a big linen trolley near the seat by the artificial plants. A dirty linen bag hanging from it is really stinky so I move to the other end of the corridor. The clothes that have come up from the general laundry are hanging on a rack in the corridor (it is taken care of by the evening shift when other tasks are done). Also carts with bed linen and towels are in the corridor. Meanwhile, one RPN student and the teacher are now taking clothes off of one rack, which they explain to me is clean clothes that have just been brought back from the laundry, and are placing them on another rack according to resident name/room number. They let me know that they then will disperse them to the correct person's bedroom to complete the task of putting away laundry.

Another field note, based on following an evening worker down the hall, expands on the effect that laundry has on the home environment: "I notice as we're walking down the hall that the wire carts, when the bags are empty, are very loud in the quiet hallway – they rattle so much with no weight in the empty bags. Surely this would disturb residents trying to sleep? It sounds like someone pushing a wire grocery cart over cobblestone."

At first glance, putting clothes on racks in the hallway seems to be an efficient way to deliver them if they are washed together in a central place, as they are in this site. Similarly, filling bins with dirty linens and pushing the bins down the hallway until they are full may seem like the safest and most time-saving way of getting rid of the soiled materials that are produced every day. However, as one resident put it, the racks make the place "look like Walmart" and some residents treat the racks that way, going "shopping" and choosing clothes for themselves from the selection. Another resident also emphasized the institutional nature of the clothes distribution system: "You never know which one is going to bring your clothes back. You know the old store racks they would hang clothes for you to go and look through? Well, they have a couple of racks like that that they hang the clothes on and then they bring them to your room because your stamp is on them. They're always on wire racks."

As this resident explains, the wire clothing racks invoke a store more than they do a homelike environment. But this approach does not only contradict the efforts to makes these places homes; it also undermines the efficiency it is intended to produce. As a worker in this home explains, "sometimes during the days when we change their clothes … some other clothes is mixed [in]. That's the big problem for us too." Trying to figure out which clothes belong to which resident can be challenging and time-consuming, taking away from other efforts to create support of the sort we seek at home.

Like the wire racks, clothing labels are intended to make the laundry process more efficient and to ensure residents' belongings are properly returned. It makes sense to label clothes, for as a UK resident observed, "I think that comes naturally to a place like this because some things are exactly the same as yours." However, we heard that in some nursing homes labelling is often delayed due to the time constraints of staff or because visitors bring gifts of unlabelled clothes, creating inefficiencies in a system based on labelling. Having to hunt down unlabelled clothing can be particularly difficult if the laundry is outsourced, as one Ontario resident explained:

> I think it's a lousy system. This is what we were going to talk with yourself and I think what my complaint was that the clothes might not come back. We don't know. I had a couple of the workers here that said, "Oh, they called us from that other hospital and said they had four or five pairs of slacks with no ID number on them." They didn't have a yellow label on them and they thought they might be mine. Well then as days went by and days went by and nobody said anything I asked again and they said, "Oh, they didn't send them over because they thought they had somebody else that might own them." So it's just a riddle.

Moreover, labelling can also limit other efficiencies. A growing number of residents die within months of entering the home and when roommates die, the remaining resident(s) often need to be moved to different rooms in order to accommodate issues such as gender, culture, or preferences for privacy. Our field notes indicate that a representative of the nurses' union in BC pointed out that "when residents move rooms it is 'a big pain' because 'you have to change the marking of the clothes, you have to change the number.' The clothing labels include the room number at this facility, causing problems when residents have to move rooms to a room with more appropriate equipment." Labels can also fall off or fade over time. Further-more, despite their obvious utility, clothing labels are not particular-ly homelike themselves, compounding the already unhomelike feel-ing of the wire racks, laundry trolleys, and soiled laundry bins. Thus the strategies devised to make sure residents get back their own be-longings may additionally undermine the attempt to make the nurs-ing home a home.

Although pushing a bin down the hallway so it can be filled as each resident is washed and dressed may save time, the smells from the soiled linens pollute the air. This pollution makes the entire place unpleasant and unsafe for workers, families, and residents. Add to this the noise pollution from the rattling carts and it is not a place like home. Indeed, noises that wake residents make more work for care providers and less comfort for residents.

Ontario was not alone in such unhomelike treatment of clothes. In Texas, for example, one site we studied had a very similar approach to the distribution of clothes and, as we indicated earlier, we rejected a site visit to another facility because the soiled laundry smell was strong as soon as we entered the front door. It even permeated the director's office. Scandinavia is not exempt from the smell problem either. A Norway field note records that the "laundry is stored in the hallways, giving a cluttered/neglected feel to the environment of the facility." How the laundry is processed in the interest of efficiency thus has larger implications for the sights, sounds, and smells of a nursing home – elements that can enhance the homelike feel of a setting or, as we saw much more frequently, not.

Balancing the need for efficiency in dealing with large amounts of laundry while creating a homelike atmosphere is no simple task. We saw alternatives, however, to the unhomelike sight of carts full of smelly laundry blocking the halls. In a Norway site, staff bring dirty linen to the dirty linen utility room directly rather than using a cart system. Similarly, in Nova Scotia the laundry worker picks up dirty clothes from individual rooms and carries them to bins out of sight. Once they are laundered, she returns them to a closet for clean clothes in the main room, where care providers pick out the clothes for the resident they are about to dress. Linens are still piled in carts, howev-er, although not stored in the hallway. They are removed at night so that the process is largely invisible to residents and families. In a German home, there is an outside door in front of two resident bedroom doors, and the clean linen can be stored just outside the actual bedroom in the space in between. Such an arrangement prevents the kind of "shopping" off the wire racks we saw in Ontario and allows residents more privacy than when clothes are stored in the main room.

When clothing is washed in the resident's room, as it was in a site we visited in Sweden, the smells of dirty laundry do not enter the hallway and there are no racks full of clothes in the hall. Not incidentally, care workers are less likely to be injured filling washing machines in a single room than they are when lifting heavy loads gathered from multiple rooms, and infections are less likely to spread. Clothes do not often get lost either. Of course, the initial cost of placing the machinery in each room is significantly higher than the initial cost of concentrating machinery in a central place, and there are implications for the division of labour. However, there are important benefits to be had in terms of helping the nursing home to sound, look, and smell more like a home.

Many of the places we visited centralized the linen laundry. This tends to be the heaviest and the most infectious of the laundry. These linens are not related to personal choice, identity, or dignity, except when they are not changed or there is insufficient supply. Moreover, they are made to withstand high heat and so are in less danger of being wrecked in the laundry process. Centralization may thus make sense for washing linens. A Swedish worker, for example, said, "I would like there to [be] central laundry on the residents' sheets for hygienic reasons. It is more hygienic and more for the working environment." It can work well for both residents and workers. However, this is not the case when the linens are collected and returned in huge hallway bins and when the centralized laundry is an isolated workplace without air or windows, as we saw in some sites. But handling clothes in a centralized laundry can undermine efforts both to make these places homes and to give residents some personal status. Clothing is more likely to go missing or be damaged in a centralized laundry, especially if that laundry is located off-site as in the case with contracting out, undermining the sense of home.

Clothes and Homes

It is not only how the halls sound, look, and smell but also how the residents look and smell that makes a place homelike. In the previous chapter, we documented the various ways families, workers, and residents told us that clothes reflect their values, their personal history, and their personal status. Clothes are also understood as an indicator of homelike care and as integral to person-centred care. In Ontario, a family member commented on the contrast with home evident in "residents sitting around and, you know, very untidy." She offered the specific example of Sam, who was an accountant. "He was very much of a perfectionist in his dress and his style at home, you know, so I guess that's why things like that bother me." Sam may have looked perfect at home but such perfection may conflict with conditions in long-term residential care.

Not all resident clothing preferences are ideal from the perspectives of safety, of what others see as appropriate, or of the practicalities of care provision. Allowing residents to choose their clothing may cause issues for monitoring and maintaining cleanliness. Our field notes at one Ontario home, for example, indicate that while some residents appeared to be able to dress themselves and choose their own clothing, it was not always clear whether residents who could choose their own clothing were being sufficiently monitored by care workers to make sure that their clothing was being regularly changed and laundered, as some wore the same items repeatedly.

Moreover, residents may select clothing that conflicts with what families perceive as appropriate. Indeed, laundry and clothes illustrate the need to balance tensions between the expectations of families and the preferences of residents. Not all of the residents' choices meet with the approval of relatives. We heard from both managers and workers that families not infrequently objected to how a resident was dressed even when the choices were those of the resident alone. Families also objected to staff choices in clothing. "Dressing up" residents can be infantilizing (Dobbs et al. 2008; Tarbox 1983), and some families told us workers sometimes dressed a resident in what the family considered culturally inappropriate or undignified ways. Dressing residents with flowers in their hair at one UK home, for example, was seen as "treating them like babies." And emphasizing gender-normative clothing may contradict a resident's identity but please the family. While we raised such questions in our interviews and sought to include these concerns in our observations, we did not uncover obvious cases – but this does not mean they do not exist. Training, managerial guidance, and cultural sensitivity combined with familiarity with the resident and family may well mitigate these concerns, but much more research is required to identify factors that separate supportive from infantilizing dressing up.

Balancing the need to support resident clothing choices that make them feel at home with the need to perform bodily care can be particularly challenging for care workers when assisting residents who are frail or physically disabled. For example, we spoke with care workers at an Ontario nursing home who had daily difficult encounters with a resident who insisted on wearing overly tight clothing that workers had to struggle to remove, causing strain injuries for the workers and pain for the resident when her clothes had to be changed. However, the alternative option of adaptive clothing can challenge residents' dignity, and can also be prohibitively expensive in requiring alterations or a whole new wardrobe. While snap closures may mean less pulling on limbs, snaps can come undone while residents move about. As one relative noted, this can lead to the undignified situation of residents appearing "half dressed" in the public spaces of the nursing home, with gaps in their clothing. Furthermore, getting preferences wrong in dressing a resident can have serious consequences for care workers, including violent outbursts from residents during the dressing process.

There is also a tension between the need to control infection and the need to protect clothing from the means of infection control. When we asked in a German site about responses on the questionnaires given regularly to residents and their families, the nurse supervisor responded: "Mostly it's concerning clothing because some clothing is not [put] away or it's ... the laundry is on the wrong temperature so it don't fit anymore." In chapter 3 we explained that the temperatures at which clothes are washed, and the chemicals used to wash them, are intended to prevent the spread of infection and ensure that linens and clothes are safe for the residents. It makes sense from a clinical perspective to wash the clothes together in a single efficient laundry where the chemicals are more easily handled in industrial machines, and to require residents to have clothes that can withstand the subsequent threat of damage from sanitizing detergents and high heat. It is particularly important when residents are incontinent or have some other health issue that requires frequent changes in clothes, or if they have an infection. Balancing the tension between the need to keep residents smelling good and to maintain sufficient sanitation, on the one hand, and creating a homelike atmosphere on the other is not easy to achieve, especially when we may have ideal notions of what constitutes a home. Homelike frequently loses out to institutional-like clothing, especially when regulations focus on sanitation.

Clothes at home are cared for in particular ways, ways that are hard to replicate in a nursing home. Consider the perspective offered by one manager, who told us that residents frequently complain that their clothing is being damaged in the wash at their nursing home: "The number of times I've been told off by somebody – 'You're washing my clothes away. You're washing them too much' – because they didn't used to. They used to take them off, fold them, and they'd wear them for more than one day." At home, a person does not necessarily wash something after wearing it once – doing so would indeed wear out our clothing quite quickly. In one's own home one has control over not only how something is washed, but also what gets washed and how often. However, in a nursing home, clothing may be much more frequently washed for a number of reasons: residents' clothing may be more often stained/soiled as their capacities decline; rules may require staff to put residents' clothing in the wash after each wear; and with shift rotation or irregular shift work, staff may not know how long a resident has been wearing their clothes. Regardless of the reasons, the need to wash clothing more frequently and to maintain nursing home sanitation contrasts with how persons generally care for clothing at home, resulting in clothing being "washed away" too soon and destabilizing the homelike quality of the setting for residents.

One way the problem is addressed, as we have seen, is by regulating the kind and amount of clothing that residents can bring with them. However, preventing people from bringing any delicate clothes into the facility or limiting their closet space also means preventing them from dressing as they would at home. This is not an uncommon way of addressing the tension, as we heard from a care worker in the UK: "Lots of care homes where I come from, no one is allowed to have

woollens and no one is allowed to have delicates." But banning delicate clothes is not the only possible response to the tension between
the need for sanitary conditions and residents' clothing choices.
Indeed, this worker told us about her prior experience to contrast it
with the current one. The laundry department of this UK nursing
home is equipped with smaller machines, like those found in one's
own home. Laundry workers could separate out the more delicate
clothing and process it separately in these machines. For the laundry
worker at this nursing home, making it possible for residents to wear
the clothes they would in their own home allows them to retain their
dignity. She saw this as a critical issue for residents and no big deal for
the laundry workers. Indeed, it gave her satisfaction to provide this
care, and she saw it as a central contribution to residents' well-being.
"So you see, these small things are very important." Although these
small things make it feel more like home, they take time and often
cost more in terms of labour, creating another tension in today's cost-
cutting world.

Moreover, a focus on getting the appropriate clothes on people
each day often conflicts with what are understood as the clinical priorities. Indeed, one Canadian doctor we interviewed used specifics
about clothing as an example of how needlessly detailed the care
plans are: "The only thing that's mandated in long-term care is the
care plan and so the care plan tends to be very long with details. You
know, 'Mrs Smith likes to wear her blue dress every Thursday before
she goes to mass. Make sure you put her little necklace on.'" For this
doctor, and for many managers and nurses we interviewed, priority
must go to clinical care, and the attention to things like clothes not
only conflicts with that focus but can also undermine it. Yet the blue
dress and necklace are what Mrs Smith wore at home, and they can
provide a means of reassuring her that the nursing home is now her
new home, providing a sense of continuity through dress. Reflecting
this approach in practice, we saw in some homes residents who were
not only dressed respectably but dressed up with clear attention to
personal detail, as if they were about to have company at home. Field
notes from a German site, for example, indicate that residents are
dressed in a range of clothing styles, and with accessories that reflected individuals' preferences:

Residents are dressed more nicely than I generally observe. They have leather shoes, dress pants, clean shirts and sweaters that do not appear worn, or stretched and I do not see track pants. They are wearing fitted, quality skirts i.e. pleated, dress pants, cardigans, and collared blouses. Clothes match, like time has been taken in the choosing of items to put together for the day. One woman has a black bead necklace as well, another a small pair of earrings, tastefully attired. Shoes are mostly leather, some with little heels or wedges. A couple of women are wearing foam bootie slippers.

Supporting residents' preferences for the full range of clothing options, from casual foam bootie slippers to fine blouses and pleated skirts, requires more work on the part of those who dress residents as well as on the part of those who wash the clothes. And it requires enough staff. Blouses and some materials may require more delicate processing, and pleated clothing such as dress pants requires ironing. In many homes we visited, ironing either is not done due to time constraints or, as we saw in chapter 2, is done on unpaid overtime and by family members.

However, in some homes workers have sufficient flexibility and resources to better support residents' clothing choices. In a UK home with an in-house laundry department and a manager determined to provide personal care, laundry workers explained, "We don't do a great deal of ironing," as most residents' clothes do not require it. However, they do offer ironing as part of the service: "I mean obviously if they need ironing, but if it doesn't need ironing we don't iron." When we inquired further, it became clear that deciding whether the clothes "need ironing" was based not solely on the fabric or cut of the clothes, but also on the preferences and previous life of the resident. "I mean, the thing is as well some people have always dressed well, some people don't bother. Some people like fancier clothes and we've got a few ladies like that." At this UK home, residents' preference to dress up in "fancier" clothing – which requires more labour – is supported by workers having the flexibility to decide and prioritize which clothes to spend more time on. This decision-making is in turn supported by workers' knowledge of residents' preferences. Knowing the residents also takes some flexibility in work organization, and at this UK home there is an explicit policy of including all workers – laundry, dietary, maintenance, etc. – as a part of the care team. This approach not only helps workers to feel included and valued, but also allows workers to tailor care to residents' individual preferences for a "fancier" appearance.

In sum, the pressure to achieve efficiencies and prevent the spread of germs along with the increasing emphasis on clinical care conflict with efforts to make these places homes and to support personal dignity. We did, however, see examples of balancing these tensions that favoured a homelike atmosphere without sacrificing safety and clinical care. Sometimes these places had more staff, sometimes the location of laundry equipment allowed more attention to dress, and sometimes the manager was committed to relational care.

Clothes for Work in Homes

Although these places are advertised as homes for residents, they are workplaces for many others and places of germ transmission for all. The tension between home and work is often visible in what staff wear and in how they deal with laundry. A bunch of people bustling around in uniforms does not make a place feel like home. Nor do people wearing latex gloves to handle clothes.

Among the twenty-five homes we visited, however, it was common for staff to wear uniforms. The reasons given for the uniforms are similar, although not always the same. Uniforms are easy to keep clean and many of the things staff do are messy. Uniforms can be more hygienic, thus reducing the risk of spreading infections. They can also provide appropriate pockets, making tasks easier, or prevent residents from grabbing clothing. Uniforms signal who is a worker and who is not, an issue when friends, volunteers, and privately paid companions are floating around the home. Moreover, when the uniforms are colour-coded they can symbolize the division of labour, telling residents and families who can do what for whom.

Practices often tended to contradict these justifications, however. Although in Sweden and Norway uniforms were washed in the workplace, in the Canadian and the US sites we visited it was common for workers to travel to and from work in their uniforms. It is difficult to see how travelling in your uniform to and from work can limit the spread of germs. In a German home we visited, the uniforms supplied by the home came in three sizes and were colour-coded by size (the largest size being yellow), signalling to others not the job category, but rather body size. This approach exemplifies how uniforms supplied by the employer can not only make the place feel institutional for residents and families but can also make the workers uncomfortable. In Sweden, our field notes suggest another way that uniforms provided by the facility are not necessarily an easy solution: "When the third [assisting nurse] arrived she was laughing and told her colleagues she was embarrassed. Why? Her clothes didn't fit. The trousers are [too] short and the t-shirt too long. They tell me that when they moved to the new building they got new clothes which they ordered in their personal size (jeans and red t-shirt or red dress). The clothes get washed at a laundry and get mixed up. People take more clothes than they actually are allowed to so there is a shortage of working clothes in the right size." So at this nursing home, the workers face the same problem as the residents in many other places: lost, ill-fitting, and inappropriate clothing.

In an Ontario home, workers had previously worn whatever they found comfortable and argued that this made the residents more comfortable as well, making it look more like home. As one care worker at this home explained, "I mean, to me, wearing your own stuff makes you unique, right? As opposed to everyone being in the same uniform. Uniqueness helps especially with the residents. Then they can identify you as opposed to like seeing you in a uniform and identifying some sort of institution. Especially for the women, they can come in with printed tops and stuff, which really makes for a more, how would I say, homey setting as opposed to an institution. I mean, the uniform really sort of institutionalizes the whole environment." As we indicated in chapter 4, the management had recently introduced colour-coded uniforms that, according to care workers, changed the environment from a "homey setting" to an institutionalized one while emphasizing hierarchy. The more flexible division of labour in the Nordic countries means such coding is not required, but uniforms were still common in the homes we studied.

We did visit homes where the workers wore what they felt was comfortable, which was often clothing that looked more like they were going to exercise class. These places, such as one home in the UK we

studied, did look less institutional than the places with uniforms, and
we did not see anyone have difficulty identifying staff, although this
place had a policy that promoted a very flexible division of labour.
Washing what workers wear on site, as they do in Norway, can also contribute to safety, but the clothes washed this way need not be uniforms.

This is not to say, however, that uniforms are uniformly problematic for all workers. Although the uniforms contradict the efforts to create a homelike atmosphere and also seem to contradict some of the
other justifications for them, we also heard from some staff that they
preferred the uniforms and all they implied. They liked the identity,
protection, and convenience that come with the uniform. The tension
is thus not easily resolved by giving workers a choice in what to wear.

The issue of protective clothing such as gloves is even more complicated. We visited homes in several countries that had containers for
latex gloves outside every room, and homes where gloves were not in
evidence in the corridors or in residents' rooms. There is no question
that gloves are often necessary for the safety of both the worker and
the resident. Placing them in easily accessible places encourages their
use when necessary and reminds workers to use them. There is also no
question that containers on the wall do not make the place look like
home and instead emphasize the clinical. Yet several homes seem to
be able to keep infections low and handle messy linens without making gloves so prominent.

In short, uniforms symbolize the workplace, as do protective items
like gloves. They also signal that clinical care is a priority and that
there is a work hierarchy. Some homes we visited have resisted uniforms and limit the use of gloves, although a significant number of
staff we talked with opposed such approaches. The places without
uniforms and gloves in boxes outside the rooms did look more homelike. Some of these were places that emphasized and followed a particular model of care, while others reflected staff preferences, supported by unions.

AUTONOMY AND RISK

Ever since the famous Whitehall study of British civil servants began
in 1967 (see Marmot et al. 1978; Marmot et al. 1991), it has been recognized that control and autonomy are critical factors in workers'

health. People are healthier when they have the right to decide and to act independently, while still taking others into account. At the same time, concern about risk is central to how governments, employers, and workers act, and this may be the basis for limits on autonomy. As Hannah-Moffat and O'Malley (2007, 2) explain, "We often participate willingly in these regimes of risk because they promise, and often deliver, greater safety and security. Yet we buy in at a cost: we allow much of our daily lives to be delimited by considerations of risk that take into account futures that are unlikely to happen to the average person." Highly publicized scandals (Lloyd et al. 2014) have reinforced concerns about risks in long-term residential care. The risks can come from the physical and social environment, from residents, and from staff without the appropriate training and supports. Balancing the concerns about safety with the benefits of autonomy is no simple task.

Resident involvement in the work of the home provides one example of the tension between autonomy and risk. Homes are usually associated with both a degree of independence and some participation in domestic labour. For women especially, doing laundry work and choosing their own clothes can make them feel at home, given that this is work most of them did at home. However, allowing residents to do this laundry and clothing work may also involve more staff time, thus putting other tasks at risk, and can create some risk to residents.

In a Swedish nursing home, the care staff strongly supported the notion that residents should do their own laundry if they can and felt this was especially the case for women: "We have a lot of women who live here, they'd love to do, absolutely, they are welcome to help with that as simple as setting the table, washing up, pick stuff and go into the laundry and fold clothes and stuff, it's good, it's employment for them too." As we pointed out in the previous chapter, in a German nursing home we visited, these women were paid modestly for doing such tasks, formally recognizing their contribution to the work of the home and providing them some control over the job. However, the majority of residents in all the homes we visited were very frail and half had some form of dementia, making it more difficult or even risky for them to do laundry. We did see some residents doing their own laundry in spite of this, albeit with some difficulty and adaptations as the field notes from a Canadian site illustrate: "A resident named 'P' comes out of the laundry room, pulling a basket of laundry with him using a device that is like an extendable gripper arm – one of those things you can use to reach something on a high shelf, or that falls behind the couch or something. He drags the laundry basket as far out of the laundry room as he can so that the door will shut, then tries to lean over far enough to lift the basket onto his lap; however he can't seem to lean forward far enough." Moreover, allowing residents to do their own laundry may mean that the clothes are not always appropriately cleaned, as field notes from this home further indicate: "The PCAs continue to chat amongst themselves and laugh at a male resident who walks down the hall with some dirty clothes on the way to the laundry room. They laugh that it is funny that he chooses to do his own laundry because he does it without soap." The lack of soap may not only mean that his clothes are dirty, but also that others using the machine may put their clothes at risk of infection.

The physical design of laundry facilities may also create risks for these frail residents. Although an Ontario care aide saw the benefit of laundry work for some residents, she was worried about the heavy laundry room door at her facility. "You look at OT [occupational therapy] and they say, 'That's a good thing. You want to keep active,' and I certainly can understand that. If you're able to, hey great, you know, if you want to." However, as she went on to say, "But like I say, some of them just aren't able to and don't have anybody to do it so I don't think it should come out of their pocket." Her concern was that laundry work was shifted to residents regardless of capacity as a way of saving money for the nursing home.

But allowing residents the autonomy to do their own laundry can address at least one clothes problem in nursing homes, if the equipment is appropriate. One resident in this nursing home took to washing his own clothes because his kept getting lost. He was pleased when they put in the laundry for residents and their families. "Then I could take them myself and go to the washing machine down the hall. I didn't trust my clothes coming back. So I started doing all my own clothes." However, he did not appreciate the heavy door. "Trying to get into the door to the laundry machines is like trying to break into Fort Knox." Furthermore, the machines here and in other homes we visited were often broken, and it was suggested that this reflected their use by residents who were not up to the task. So while the home did have a laundry room that was available for residents to use, the design made such independent action less likely and riskier.

Allowing residents control over what they wear can support independence and individual identity, as we explored in chapter 4. A UK care assistant in a home where the model supported resident autonomy offered the following example, where residents choose what to wear and when:

> Or he might want to put [his] pyjamas on and leave his pyjamas on all day because you also find that you get them dressed and they go and get undressed again and change. I think he wore – was it – Mary's pink trousers one day because that's how [he] felt. He just wants to wear somebody else's clothes. I mean, it was quite comical but to him he was fine. We were, "He's got Mary's clothes on," but you try and take it off him he's going to [be unhappy] ... If he's got a pink top on or pink trousers and somebody else's shoes, it doesn't matter. Obviously when they're running around naked and what have you you've got to, you know, dress them. But nine times out of ten they're able just to live their life the way they want and I think it makes a difference when you haven't got "Sit down and have your dinner," you know.

A family member in this residence stressed how important such options are, remarking, "I think that's why the home works, because it is their home at the end of the day."

However, allowing residents this autonomy can also constitute a risk. In some other jurisdictions, regulations do not allow pyjamas in the communal spaces, and we heard from families that they objected to residents not "being properly dressed." Moreover, residents' choices often did not fit with notions of well-organized clinical care and could even mean negative marks in an inspection report. Dragging pant legs may constitute a trip hazard and women's shoes with heels can mean falls. Similarly, families may choose clothes that are too hard to put on or that require the sort of careful handling not possible in a nursing home.

Bibs, or "clothing protectors" as they are called in some nursing homes, offer another example of a contradiction between supporting independence and the need to avoid the risks of dirty clothing, more laundry, and the need to change clothes that have food spilled all over them. On the one hand, many residents have difficulty with eating, and this difficulty often results in a mess on their clothes, especially when there are not enough staff to help them eat. This either means a change in clothes or leaving residents in messy ones, something not often seen as a reasonable option given the risk to residents' dignity, as well as to the perceptions of family, workers, or inspectors that residents are being neglected. Bibs are a way of avoiding the mess, but they also do not look very dignified, and they signal dependence in alluding to childhood. And when they are made of thin blue plastic, as we saw in one UK home that was privately owned, they look very institutional.

Some homes we studied tried hard to handle this tension in innovative ways. Partly as a result of complaints from family members, a Vancouver home allows residents the choice of whether or not to wear a bib and take their chances on a mess. In a Nova Scotia home, the workers bought apron-like bibs that were made out of material that matched a local tartan, which from our perspective at least looked more "adult" and dignified compared to plastic.

Tensions around autonomy and risk are not restricted to residents and families. There are also tensions around the extent to which workers have control over what they do, or when and how they do it. Especially in Canada, licensing and other regulations define scope of practice in ways that limit who can do what in a nursing home. Those defined as unregulated workers are often restricted in terms of what they can do with and for residents. They are also at the bottom of a hierarchy, which often means they have little formal capacity to make decisions about their work (Day 2014). The restrictions, and their place at the bottom of the hierarchy, are justified on the basis of lack of training and the need for safety. The laundry is done by such workers, and most residents are dressed by them as well. Moreover, worker autonomy needs to be balanced with management's need to maintain some coordination and control.

Yet there are ways to balance this tension to allow some autonomy while limiting risk. We saw and heard from workers who do laundry and are able to make decisions that shape their work in beneficial ways. In Norway, for example, a worker explained that it was the right to decide that made the work rewarding: "I like it very much espe-cially that we are very much in charge of our own work and I am responsible for making the shift lists, which are made on a six-week basis, alternates every six weeks ... For my group there's seven people and I make the shift for those seven people for every six weeks. So within our group we decide who is doing what when. Also for holidays it's our job to sort out who works when and make it fair. So we collaborate on that to make it reasonable and fair." In Sweden too, workers talked about their independence and right to decide: "For example, I have responsibilities in the laundry room, then I can say I'm tired today and ... you can take the laundry room, it's perfectly okay to change and do like this." It was even possible in Canada for such workers to have some independence and to talk with residents. As a UK worker put it: "If someone was upset you wouldn't just walk by, would you? You would sit with them even if you're not a carer." In all these instances, the risk of autonomy is limited by the teamwork that characterizes these homes and by managerial understanding of how important contact with residents is for workers. Working across occupational boundaries can mean teaching, supporting, and watch-ing each other, thus helping to both prevent and deal with risk.

In short, there are tensions between autonomy and risk, but we saw multiple strategies for shifting the balance towards autonomy without risking further risk. Managers can make a difference when they begin with the assumption that all workers need to interact with residents, that teamwork can help ensure safety, and that adequate staffing pro-motes fewer risks.

COMMUNITIES AND INDIVIDUALS

Although the tensions around autonomy are primarily about capaci-ties and risk, independence is also circumscribed by the tension between individuals and community. Although facilities are fre-quently promoted as homes, they are also communal spaces. A com-munal environment lends itself to the possibilities for sharing, sup-port, and teamwork. At the same time, living collectively necessarily involves tensions, and such tensions are intensified when the residents are frail and often have dementia, when women significantly out-number men as both residents and care providers, and when cultures or classes clash. Some of these tensions are evident when it comes to clothes.

Unlike care in the private home, the communal setting of the nursing home offers the possibility for staff to work alongside and support each other, presenting the opportunity for teamwork and shared learning. We saw many examples of such supportive teamwork, especially in those sites where there was a limited division of labour, some autonomy for all staff, and enough staff to create reasonable workloads. Even amidst heavy workloads and expanding job roles, getting through the laundry work is more feasible if working together as a team is possible. For example, a care worker at an Ontario home explained the teamwork system she and her fellow assistive personnel had developed for sorting the clothes together:

> We all work together. We all sort the clothes together. We sort all the socks together. We leave it for evening … We say, "Hey. Enough is enough. We're not going to sort it and start putting it away now." You just start doing that and then someone down there wants something. But we work as a team and that kind of helps for the end of the day saying okay, you know, you and the other person, you did what you could for the day. We're not machines. We're not robots. Sometimes they expect you to be but I mean come on.

At this home, assistive personnel had been reassigned the job of sorting laundry when the home removed its in-house laundry services. As we saw in chapter 2, this downloading of tasks adds to their workload; however, workers have devised a strategy for sorting the clothes as a team at night, when the floor is comparatively less busy and workers are less frequently called away to assist residents. Working as a team and rearranging the work helps them to feel, at the end of day, that they "did what they could" despite a heavy workload.

However, a variety of factors can shift the balance against teamwork and against the benefits of teamwork. One we have already explored is the detailed division of labour and regulations designed to ensure that each worker has the necessary skills and appropriate authority. But it can also divide staff from each other. As a UK worker put it: "Some places it's like laundry is laundry. Housekeeping is housekeeping. No mix. All very, very separate." This worker was talking about her previous experience, contrasting it to her current workplace where all workers were expected to do what needed to be done, with direct clinical care the only exception. She far preferred her current place because she could engage with residents and be part of the team in this community. She also felt it worked better for the residents.

Another factor shifting the balance is the contracting out of services. It is hard to have teams when you have different employers with different rules that also mean different degrees of autonomy. One worker in BC explained how the efforts to save money and increase efficiency through contracting out undermined teams: "Our dietary and laundry and housekeeping departments were privatized and the staff in those departments were given a pink slip. Their job was discontinued and I think they were given the option of retraining for [the] nursing department or applying to the company that was provided. Most of the staff left but a few staff stayed on and a few of the staff in dietary or laundry or what have you, they did retrain and become care aides where they were working in the kitchen or that kind of thing." A cleaner at the same site who also did laundry on occasion talked about how with privatization she was continually moved around in ways that meant she no longer knew the staff or the residents. Other cost-cutting measures, such as the pressure to complete tasks as quickly as possible, can create tensions among staff that undermine teamwork. We saw this kind of tension arise frequently when a bell rang, with workers arguing over who was too busy and whose job it was to answer. We also saw workers refuse one another's requests for assistance on similar grounds. Unions can help resist both privatization and cost-cutting, but have often done so by emphasizing the detailed division of labour in order to prevent employers from co-opting teamwork as a means of increasing workloads.

Communities also offer possibilities for support and sharing among families and residents. Take the example of clothing offered to an Ontario woman who took much of the responsibility for her grandmother who lived in the nursing home: "There was one staff member that gave my grandmother a top because my grandmother really liked it. But it didn't have a name tag on it. They didn't know who it belonged to. So it was going to go in a box to go either in the garbage or to like a place like Sally Ann's or Salvation Army or something like that." Connection and collaboration between workers and relatives can be beneficial, especially for residents with limited finances. This woman wanted to share in return, giving back to those in need in the community of her grandmother's nursing home. "I brought in a comforter that was given to me and wasn't in use with that family anymore but it was a really nice comforter. And I didn't have any use for it because I've got too many of them. And I knew my grandmother didn't need it, so I asked if I could bring it in just to give to the home to give to someone who needed it and they were able to do that. They put the person's name on it and that person now has it because they were in need of it." Being able to help out in this way made her feel like she was contributing to the home and helping to fulfill residents' needs. Furthermore, in making such an offer, she was taking gender and workers' knowledge into account: "You know, like find a home for this item knowing that it was good quality, it was pretty so it would be more for a female than a male. And they knew exactly who to give it to as soon as I brought it in, exactly the person for it ... Like the staff know the residents. They knew exactly who they wanted to give it to, who needed it." She was far from alone in providing such support especially for those she saw as poor. Another Ontario woman, for example, said: "Like I've given bags of clothes. Always have, because the thing is a lot of the people who live here don't have family members and they don't have extra money for clothing and stuff."

Such sharing in the nursing home community can contribute to the dignity and comfort of residents while adding little cost to the residence. It may mean that those who have no family and are poor are provided with essential clothing, as we were told in a Texas home where unclaimed lost-and-found items are donated to residents in need. At this particular home, as we learned in our tour, there are many in need of such communal support: "We then toured the laundry facilities (3 large industrial machines, one of which was broken) and viewed a 'lost and found' clothing bin for the clothes of departed residents which had not been claimed. If not picked up by relatives within a certain period of time, these clothes would be donated to current residents who needed them (underscoring the significantly poor Medicaid proportion of the clientele)." However, such giving and sharing is not without tensions. Offering clothing raises questions about privacy, ownership, class, and cultural preference: "[A worker] asked me if it was okay if she gave it to my nanny ... Like they have to ask before they give. A family member has to be asked, whether it be the resident or a family member of the resident, before it gets put in their room or gets labelled with their name on it to be put into their room. You can't just put something into the room." In this home, the management decided workers should not be involved in redistributing clothes in this way. This decision came in part because management feared some family members would complain based on their class or cultural backgrounds. There was also a concern that a family may be offended at seeing their relative dressed in the clothes of a dead person. Being dressed in hand-me-downs can also invoke the stigma of charity.

This conflict between managerial concerns and workers' strategies for making sure that residents have enough clothing illustrates the tension between community and individuals. On the one hand, nursing homes have the potential to promote sharing and redistribution of resources, which can support resident dignity in making sure that everyone has enough appropriate clothes to wear. At the same time, this approach raises concerns over individual dignity and may incite individual conflict, presenting a barrier to the full benefits of communal life.

Communal places can be sources of other tensions among residents. As we have seen, clothes go missing sometimes because others take them off the clean clothes racks and claim them as their own. We heard residents accuse each other of stealing their clothes, even out of their rooms, and family members upset because they saw another woman wearing, for example, their mother's sweater. We heard families complain about the failure to dress their relative or store their clothes in a way that ensured privacy. Allowing and paying workers to purchase clothes for those going without and installing washing machines in each room can help resolve some of these tensions.

In short, while communities may encourage sharing, support, and teamwork, they also raise concerns about individual privacy, and conditions can limit the possibilities for teamwork. Unions and managers, in seeking to protect workers or respond to family concerns, may shift the balance to the individual in ways that may limit some benefits of community.

SHORT- AND LONG-TERM STRATEGIES

A contradiction we heard about repeatedly was the one between short-term strategies designed to save money and the long-term costs that can result. Budgets tend to be assigned on a yearly basis, making longer-term planning difficult. In many places, the budgets are also assigned to specific categories, so savings in one category can mean higher costs in another.

A telling example comes from a manager in an Ontario home who studied the use of slider sheets in their complex care unit and became convinced that they would be more efficient. As she explained, it was difficult to convince long-term care administrators to use the slider sheets "because it was very expensive initially, right? It was an extra thing you had to go buy ... and somebody had to wash them." The sliders would mean initial expenditures not only on purchasing them but also perhaps on laundry. But she knew money could be saved in the long-term by making the investment, and that benefits could be had for the workplace as a whole. She started her campaign by using the slider sheet in palliative care because workers experienced high injury rates there and she wanted to demonstrate the impact on those rates. "Our data showed that our injuries went down, so then we presented [the proposal for slider sheets purchase]. It felt better [that] we had data."

Although this home is committed to basing change on evidence and on evidence that takes into account all the costs, including injuries, funding formulas focused on the short term often limit actions based on evidence. For the Ontario manager, "one of the challenges we had with long-term care with anything we do is that any prevention strategies we put in place, especially if it's equipment oriented, there's a cost associated with that so a lot of what will be happening is baby steps, you know, trial the product, demonstrate its value, get the buy-in from there. And certainly we find in long-term care it's even more challenging because budgets are a lot narrower, they're a lot tighter, and there's less flexibility often to bring new equipment on board specifically in long-term care." This Ontario manager found that investment in slider sheets, where the longer-term savings are not initially apparent, was a "hard sell," even from a cost-savings perspective. "It took us at least a year or more before they decided that yes, we would at least trial this product with you and then see who else wants it." Once the trial was approved, she involved the staff in the trial process and then used the evidence to convince others that the product made sense not only in terms of the direct costs of laundry but also in the indirect costs of injuries: "We were fortunate that the feedback we got from staff in doing the trial plus the reduction of injury rates both supported what we're looking at here. So I think overall our soft tissue injuries, you know, the general wear-and-tear types of injuries, plus the backs, the necks, and everything else, we reduced that by about 45 per cent on this one unit through implementing this product." From the perspective of management, a decrease in injuries also represents cost savings over the long term: fewer workers will be off on leave, and less compensation will be paid. So while slider sheets have a high initial purchase cost, the long-term savings are located in reducing injury rates as well as in overall laundry costs, but both are difficult to see in the short term.

Introducing slider sheets at this home not only required staff involvement in the trials but also training and continuing engagement of staff, as this manager explained. "And of course whenever you implement it staff have to get used to it. You have to provide training for it. We have to make sure, you know, this is ongoing support that's always going to be there." Support also came from residents, as she observed:

We also have to look at benefits for the clients themselves because they are our clients. We are a service-based industry so a lot of the feedback from the clients is also positive as well. They feel that it's easier on them. You know, it's more dignified for them to be using this than having three or four staff grab them and pull them up in bed and stuff like that as opposed to using two of them with this product. And it's always on the bed as well so it's always available to be used 24/7. So that's probably more of a more recent large-scale kind of example I can give you, but it's the same process that we have in place for small things.

But funding formulas are not the only barrier to developing long-term strategies when policies and processes are based on cutting short-term costs. There are also limits imposed by supply companies, by work processes, and by the need to coordinate with other institutions, as this manager explains. In order to be able to purchase the sliders and get them washed, she had to work with other institutions such as the hospitals, the laundry companies, and government policies. "From their point of view it all comes down to dollars and cents, what's the return going to be, what are other organizations going to be looking for?"

The long-term investment in slider sheets enhanced the care of the home by making the transfer process more dignified for residents – a benefit impossible to capture in funding formulas. The experience with slider sheets at this home thus illustrates the tension between the focus on short-term costs that are narrowly defined and longer-term savings in terms of direct and indirect costs.

Contracting out provides a contrary example based on similar pressures. Having a private-sector company do the laundry looks like it can save money and make budgets look better in the short term. The lower cost is assumed to be based on the greater efficiency of for-profit concerns compared to public ones: their economies of scale and their lower wages. However, the evidence (Grant, Pandey, and Townsend 2014; Public Services International Research Unit 2014) indicates that these companies also often start raising prices after they have secured the first contract. Once homes get rid of their laundry machines, laundry rooms, and laundry staff, it is too expensive to change their minds. Investing in new machines would wreck the short-term budgets.

Strategies that link changes across the nursing home are easier when homes have stable and adequate funding, because money can be shifted to ensure benefits in the long run. Long-term planning that takes into account the full range of direct and indirect costs is also more possible when these budgets are set for several years. However, if the savings go to profit rather than care, the benefits to residents, workers, and families are likely to be limited. The biggest contradiction is that the focus on cost savings ends up costing more in the long run – not only in terms of dollars and cents, but also in terms of care and working conditions.

CONCLUSIONS

Feminist political economy draws our attention to contradictions and tensions, only some of which we have explored here through laundry and clothing in the nursing homes of our study. The overarching contradictions are those between clinical and social care, and those between neo-liberal cost-cutting strategies and ensuring quality care. Making these places home is complicated by the growing demand for clinical skills as a result of the changing needs of residents. Autonomy for both residents and workers is shaped by the priority given to clinical concerns and by governments prioritizing safety. Living communally necessarily puts limits on individuals' spaces and choices but also has benefits resulting from sharing work, resources, and social life.

But we saw examples of ways to address these tensions, to balance them in ways that support both staff and residents. Understanding that clothes and laundry are central to creating a homelike atmosphere is the starting point in designing nursing homes and work organization that integrate the labour and the equipment seamlessly in care practices. Autonomy supported by teams and adequate staffing can help mitigate risks. Emphasizing and supporting the communal aspects of nursing-home living can be done in ways that still respect individual values and privacy.

6

Conclusions

We did not start our major research project with a focus on laundry and clothing. We did, however, begin with an assumption based in feminist political economy – that the entire range of paid and unpaid work counts, as do the relationships among these various kinds of work. It was our interviews and observations that led us to focus on laundry and clothing as a way into exploring larger questions about work and care in nursing homes. Residents, families, and workers all identified laundry and clothes as critical to care. Our observations confirmed this as we smelled and viewed piles of soiled laundry or recognized their absence; as we saw residents dressed with dignity and residents deprived of their dignity because of their dress or undress.

Our feminist political economy also led us to look at the larger context, initially through analytically mapping the six different countries involved. It became clear that the nature of the welfare state matters, as it determines investment, ownership, and accountability structures as well as notions about the right to care. The higher investment in public nursing homes evident in the social democratic countries reflected their commitment both to social rights and to the elderly. This commitment was reflected in the higher staffing levels, the better working conditions, and the physical design of the nursing homes that made laundry and clothing more integral to care, at least in comparison to the UK, the US, and Canada. Insurance investment in corporatist Germany, combined with funding for apprentices, also contributed to higher staffing levels. These countries also devoted less time to reporting, which allowed more time for care, greater flexibility in the division of labour, and more teamwork. The social democratic countries relied more on trust and local decision-making compared to the North American jurisdictions. There were also differences in what is understood as work that deserves pay. In Norway, when care workers go out to purchase clothes for residents in need their time is paid, and when residents in Germany do dishes or laundry, there is some compensation to acknowledge the contributions of this work to the functioning of the home.

At the same time, neo-liberal restructuring strategies that emphasize markets, fewer welfare provisions, and more individual responsibility have become more common in all of these countries. To varying degrees in the countries we included in our project, governments have turned to the private, for-profit sector to provide service delivery and models for management. Research indicates that in health services, privatization in various forms tends to increase cost in the long run while also undermining the quality of care (Harrington 2013; McGregor and Ronald 2011) and shifting the labour from paid to unpaid work. Combined with the emphasis on clinical concerns in the wake of privatization strategies that mean admission is restricted to those with complex care needs, the result is too often a focus on tasks and speed rather than on care.

Concentrating on clothing and laundry allowed us to explore how variations among and within jurisdictions in relation to privatization play out in practice. In one Swedish home, laundry done not only on site but also in individual rooms allowed residents more choices in terms of their clothes and workers more variety as well as more control over tasks. However, creeping privatization in this site is reducing staffing levels in ways that speed up the work while limiting clothing options for both residents and workers. In a Canadian home, privatization of laundry services meant clothing options were restricted and clothes were often lost or destroyed. Laundry workers had little contact with individual residents while assistive personnel spent more time sorting clothes returned from the centralized laundry. However, centralized laundry services for sheets and towels did contribute to infection control and did produce some efficiencies, although we did not see what it meant for workers at the centralized sites.

Alongside a growing reliance on the for-profit sector and its methods is a growing reliance on accountability through data recording.

Researchers in our project (Lloyd et al. 2014) have shown how this move toward an auditing culture has gained prominence with the exposure of scandals linked to market approaches in public services. While this counting can help improve some aspects of care, our research on auditing in relation to clothes and laundry suggests that it often takes time away from care and reduces worker autonomy without substantially improving quality. It also serves to reinforce hierarchies that undermine teamwork, because only some people are allowed to input the data. This emphasis on recording and reporting in detail on tasks was much more common in the North American sites we visited. Yet we saw no visible evidence of better outcomes in dress or laundry in these sites compared to those in Germany, Norway, or Sweden. Indeed, we were more impressed with the way people were dressed in those countries without detailed auditing, observing more residents looking "dressed for company." Nor did the evidence we collected on infection rates suggest that infection control was better in North America, even though the residents are similar.

Work organization has long been a focus of feminist political economy, a focus that recognizes that it is not only the employers but also the workers who shape this organization. We saw two basic kinds of work organization in the sites we visited: a detailed division of labour and a flexible division of labour. There can be good reasons to have a detailed division of labour. It can help ensure everyone has the skills they need and can determine who is responsible for what. Clinical skills have become increasingly important as the resident population has become increasingly medically complex, and the skills to manage this medically complex care require considerable training. As the specific clinical needs of residents increase, so does the pressure to ensure staff have clinical skills that are recognized by licensing bodies. A clear division of labour can thus help protect both workers and residents. Signalled by distinct uniforms, residents and families can more easily tell who can do what. Especially in North America where they face strong privatization strategies, unions often support a clear division of labour because it allows them to defend the specific rights of particular job categories in relation to others and to limit multitasking that can mean workers are exploited.

A clear division of labour may also offer workers a path into employment and training because it may create a career ladder. In the UK we were told that laundry work offered those who had little formal training a way into careers in long-term care. A worker we interviewed explained that she received training for a wide range of laundry issues. The training either happened during her paid work time or was paid for if she came in for training on her days off. Once she was trained for this job and had been working in it for a while, she had the opportunity to move into other occupational categories. In Norway, laundry work could serve as an entry point for foreigners who did not pass the language test, giving them some opportunity to improve and putting them in a position to move into other work. In both cases, the detailed division of labour made such moves possible, although Norway especially has a much more fluid division of labour than is the case in North America.

However, a detailed division of labour can also mean that the priority goes to clinical care, and that non-medical aspects of care such as laundry and clothes are seen primarily in terms of infection control rather than as central to dignity. We saw a more flexible division of labour leading to more integrated care for residents and fewer clothes lost, as well as more opportunity for building relations with residents and with other workers. Those designated as doing more of the laundry and cleaning work benefited from having a range of tasks and from being included as part of the care team, especially in the social democratic countries. The absence of colour-coded uniforms indicating rank contributed to the sense of teamwork and the notion that "we all pitch in to do the work." Too often, though, under the growing pressure in all countries to save money by for-profit means, flexibility simply meant adding to the tasks of those already overburdened, and expanding the work in ways that ignored many of the skills involved in the labour. This included the family members and especially the women relatives, who were expected to fill in the gaps in laundry and clothes care. This analysis took us back to the larger context of restructuring and reinforced our understanding of the work, and assumptions about the work, as gendered.

The feminist in feminist political economy implies the recognition that gender is integral to the social structure, embedded in the way things work and in the ways they are understood to work. Gender is understood as a social relation characterized by power inequalities as well as by variations across and within specific groups. In spite of these variations, there are obvious dominant patterns. Domestic labour and care work have long been done primarily by women in all the countries we visited and there remains an assumption that this is work any woman can do by virtue of being a woman. Although there are more men now doing this work, the overwhelming majority of those paid to do this labour in long-term residential care are women. Women also do most of the unpaid labour of care work and, especially in North America, this unpaid work is increasing as the care gap grows. In all of the countries we visited, more of the paid laundry and clothing work is done by those who are immigrants and/or from racialized groups. Especially when there is a detailed division of labour, the workers tend to be crowded into the lowest rungs in the hierarchy.

In general, the work of dressing and undressing and of washing, drying, and sorting clothes has been viewed as unskilled. The notion that the work is unskilled is evident in the very limited training provided for laundry workers in most of the countries involved in this project, and the assumption of unskilled work provides a basis for the expansion of tasks described above. Training for women doing the laundry and clothing work was often seen as unnecessary, because they are women. Assistive personnel do receive more formal training and some of it focuses on clothes, but far less attention in training is paid to the importance of clothes in dignity than to clinical aspects of care. However, Germany and Norway especially are increasingly emphasizing training for assistive personnel and doing so in a way that recognizes the skills involved.

When training is provided to laundry workers, it tends to focus on infection control and obvious health hazards of the sort usually associated with the labour of men. Laundry workers and assistive personnel do receive training in how to avoid risks to their backs, and some equipment helps reduce such risks when residents are being dressed or when laundry is being moved. However, feminist political economy draws our attention to the hidden hazards of work done primarily by women, especially to those hazards that have a cumulative effect or that are influenced by the broader conditions of work. Lack of control over their own time and tasks, lack of job security, lack of respect, lack of equipment, lack of a healthy work space, lack of involvement in teams, lack of adequate compensation, and lack of time can both create hazards and limit workers' ability to apply their training. We saw these forms of structural violence in many sites (Armstrong et al. 2011). We also were told by workers about the more direct forms of violence they faced on a daily basis, such as physical violence and racism. Just as disturbing were reports that this violence, as well as other hazards, was often not taken seriously or was blamed on the workers. These conditions show up in the very high rates of absences in many of the homes we visited. Nevertheless, we saw homes that kept absences lower by implementing strategies such as supporting teams and job rotation, keeping their own rosters of part-time staff, offering career ladders, and providing both equipment and the time to use the equipment. Higher staffing levels were also critical, helping to explain the lower levels of violence in Sweden and Norway. Such strategies not only help reduce absences; they also help ensure continuity of care and thus promote care as a relationship that can be rewarding for both residents and workers.

We saw other promising practices: ones that promote care as a relationship and create conditions that allow workers to expand their skills in ways that make it more possible to treat both residents and workers with dignity and respect. For families, residents, and workers we talked with and observed, clothes are an indicator of dignity and respect. Our chapter on taking care is testimony to the strategies, big and small, that can make life worth living for residents, families, and workers. Unfortunately, regulations, funding, work organization, the search for profit or for cost savings, and assumptions about the value of clothes and laundry, along with other pressures, often make it difficult to take this kind of care.

Finally, our feminist political economy teaches us to look for tensions and contradictions. From this perspective, there is often no simple solution, and sometimes efforts to address these tensions produce new ones. The overarching tension in long-term care is between making these places homes and making them medical facilities. Combined with auditing practices and regulations that prioritize safety over risk, this tension increases as the complexity of care rises and is reinforced by the priority given to medical care. The tension between home and medical service is linked to that between the individual and the community. A right to privacy and individual resident control frequently collides with some invasion of privacy, collective activity, and the safety measures required in communal facilities. Moreover, the emphasis on short-term strategies to address current crises and funding regulations can undermine longer-term approaches that could help save money and promote care. Such tensions, we argue, cannot be eliminated: they can only be balanced. The tendency to place the emphasis on clinical care and the short term was particularly evident in North America, as was the emphasis on control and safety over privacy. The result too often is further marginalization of clothes and laundry work and workers. The result is too often the institutionalization of residents, evident when they are wearing those similar, easy-to-wash clothes or when they are simply draped in a blanket while they are wheeled to their bath on a chair piled with those clothes.

Workers have collectively and individually resisted their conditions and the ways these tensions are balanced. There are, though, some tensions and contradictions in their forms of resistance. Most obvious is taking on extra work such as bringing laundry home in order to ensure residents "look good." This kind of taking care does enhance dignity while providing workers with a sense of satisfaction, but it does not pressure employers to address the care gap. Less obvious are personal strategies such as paying a physiotherapist to help deal with hazardous laundry work. This too means the individual can experience better health but conditions do not change.

Because our project involved research in six different countries, we were able to identify some critical factors that promote taking care, which we summarize below. These are ideas worth sharing, although they have to be adapted to particular contexts.

First, public or at least non-profit ownership of the nursing home, combined with adequate funding and staffing, is an essential condition to allow a focus on taking care. When profit is the motive, quality declines, and when services are contracted out it is very hard to provide integrated care or to develop personal relationships among staff, resident, and families.

Second, and related to the first, a flexible division of labour often promotes teamwork as well as more integrated and safer care. However, this is the case only if it does not mean a lack of training or heavier workloads. Otherwise, flexibility can mean exploitation that undermines the care relationship and people providing care for which they are not trained.

Third, training is required to make work safe for staff and residents. Such training needs to recognize the skills involved and the need for appropriate equipment that promotes a homelike, clean, and smell-free atmosphere. Yet training alone is insufficient to address the full range of conditions that make the work precarious. This requires as a starting point consultation with those who do the work, and understanding and contextualizing their experiences.

Fourth, training and working in teams can help reduce risks to residents and staff. But focusing on risks can limit autonomy for residents, staff, and families while some relative autonomy can help put life into years for both residents and staff.

Fifth, physical design is critical to care, to safety, and to a homelike environment. In that physical design, it is important to think about sights and smells as well as about the social relations of those who do the laundry and clothing work. Again, consulting those who do the work is a place to start.

Sixth, detailed regulations may serve to limit rather than promote taking care. Detailed regulations can limit autonomy for management, staff, residents, and families without ensuring accountability while trust can be built through regular, non-punitive interactions with inspectors.

Seventh, and related to the regulations, is the difference a creative manager can make, especially if they are willing to push the boundaries of the regulations. Some of the creative managers we saw followed a model such as the Eden Alternative or Dementia Care Matters, while others simply applied strategies they understood as promoting care as a relationship that involved the entire staff. These formal models, though, can become institutionalized in ways that can make them too rigid.

Eighth, relational care requires continuity in staff and opportunities for all staff to interact with residents.

Ninth, unions matter and can provide critical protections for workers and job security that promotes continuity of care. However, their ability to protect workers can be undermined by state privatization strategies and government acceptance of such policies as zero-hour contracts or gendered worker compensation criteria.

Tenth, medical care needs to be balanced with social care. Doing so requires paying attention to clothes and laundry and recognizing the role they play in personal dignity and social interaction.

We found these conditions most often in the social democratic states and least often in the liberal democratic ones. We are worried, though, that even in the social democratic states the conditions of work are leading to conditions of care that mean clothes and laundry are understood neither as indicators of care nor as central to taking care. The lessons we have learned from examining this often-overlooked and seemingly mundane feature of life and labour in nursing homes may serve as a warning as well as inspiration for promising alternatives.

APPENDICES

Project Methodology*

Re-imagining Long-Term Residential Care was designed as a rapid site-switching ethnography, a unique method designed specifically to fit the project's overarching purpose of searching for promising practices in LTRC using a feminist political economy lens. Throughout the project's seven-year duration, this method was applied in site visits to LTRC homes across six countries corresponding to Esping-Andersen's (1990) typology of welfare regimes in a capitalist economic system: Canada, the US, and the UK representing a liberal welfare regime (characterized by increasing marketization, privatization, and inequity in care provision and access), Norway and Sweden representing a social democratic welfare regime (characterized by a universalist approach to care), and Germany representing a conservative welfare regime (characterized by a mix of social insurance care models). The rapid site-switching ethnographic methodology of the Re-imagining LTRC project was collectively developed over time by the project's diverse array of participants, drawing on the research efforts, expertise, and experiences of the project's research team as well as being grounded in the existing methodological literature on two types of ethnographic approaches: rapid ethnography and team ethnography.

Rapid ethnography shares many of the same techniques that have made traditional ethnography a useful approach for studying life and labour in LTRC settings. Like traditional ethnography, rapid ethnography involves multi-method collection of data, including archival

*This description of the methodology relies heavily on the methodology chapter of Day (2014).

research, surveys, participant observation in the field, interviewing, and reflexive analysis. The goal of this multi-method approach is to "collect sufficiently *complex* descriptions" of the site or case under study (Baines and Cunningham 2011, 74), providing richly detailed data on both the setting and its context. The complexities observed in ethnographic fieldwork are particularly useful for understanding both the processes of care and the processes of work in LTRC, as the level of detail produced in fieldwork can be used to "generate new theoretical concepts, identify the steps in a particular social process, reveal the organizational principles of social groupings, identify explanatory mechanisms in social dynamics, and link these issues to broader theoretical frames of understanding" (Puddephatt, Shaffir, and Kleinknecht 2009, 1–2). By participating in, or "getting close to" (Emerson, Fretz, and Shaw 2011, 2), the everyday/every-night routines of LTRC homes, researchers have used ethnographic techniques to produce complex understandings of care and work in LTRC (Bland 2005; Bland 2007; DeForge et al. 2011; Diamond 1986; Diamond 1992; Foner 1994; Gubrium 1975; Harbers, Mol, and Stollmeyer 2002; Lopez 2006a; Lopez 2006b; Lopez 2007; McColgan 2005; Savishinsky 1991).

In contrast to the traditional ethnographic methods used in prior studies of LTRC, rapid ethnography is more focused in scope, takes place over a shorter timeframe, and is conducted using a multi-researcher design. In rapid ethnography, both observations and interviews in the field are conducted with a purposive approach, focusing on particular key actors, themes, or questions of interest (Wolcott 2008). Having a clearly defined and focused purpose to the research is thus a crucial first step in identifying the variables relevant to the project's research question and guiding theory (Handwerker 2001). In the case of the Re-imagining LTRC project, this required considerable preliminary efforts to identify the key areas of interest, resulting in four fields of inquiry: approaches to care, financing and ownership, work organization, and accountability. From a feminist political economy perspective, exploring these fields additionally required initial extensive mapping of the broader social, political, economic, and historical contexts of LTRC within and across the international sites of the study.

While traditional ethnography often takes place over an extended period of months or even years, rapid ethnography – as the name would suggest – takes place over a much shorter time frame. Gathering background information on the site of study in the form of key informant interviews and textual/electronic artifacts from the site is thus essential in order to focus attention during fieldwork on the "important activities" of interest (Millen 2000, 281) – i.e., those activities that are most directly relevant to the research question. This focused approach makes rapid ethnography particularly useful for research questions that, as in the Re-imagining LTRC project, are intended to explore "the intersection of policy and practice" by contextualizing micro-level experiences within broader macro-level policies, processes, and patterns (Baines and Cunningham 2011, 77). The project was unique in the large size and international, interdisciplinary scope of the team as well as in the extent to which the entire team participated in continually refining and revising the methodology throughout the study.

The shorter time frame and focused approach of rapid ethnography are particularly useful for a project as large in scale as Re-imagining LTRC, and these features were central to the project's rapid site-switching methodology. After considerable discussion, the team decided to base site selection primarily on key informant interviews. We interviewed individuals from community organizations, unions, and government to seek their advice on where to look for promising practices and why they would recommend these nursing homes. We also consulted inspection and other reports on quality. We then approached individual homes to ask permission, based on our local knowledge and visits to the recommended locations.

Ethics approval was received from York University, the host institution; from individual homes where systems were in place; and from the universities of individual team members when this was required. Although many homes indicated they would be happy to be identified, we have made every effort to keep the names of the sites confidential. Any resident names provided in field notes are pseudonyms.

Prior to conducting on-site fieldwork, the following background documents were gathered from each LTRC home identified as a participating site:

a. The resident care policy
b. The resident bill of rights and/or facility mission statement
c. Materials on the facility's care philosophy
d. Orientation guides for new staff hires and volunteers
e. Orientation materials for new residents and/or family members of residents
f. Floor plans of the residence as a whole, including room layouts and outdoor spaces
g. Policy and procedure manuals for all types of staff
h. Collective agreements for all unionized staff types
i. Training and educational materials for all types of staff and volunteers
j. Job descriptions for all staff types (i.e., tasks and responsibilities)
k. A chart of the facility's organization and management
l. Workplace health and safety promotion materials (manuals and training documents)
m. Health and Safety Committee documents
n. Detailed information on residents: their acuity, case mix, demographic characteristics
o. Detailed information on staff: training and accreditation, number of staff by type, demographics of staff, turnover rates, absence/injury rates
p. Resident and Family Council policies
q. Other: any documents/materials relating to the facility's organizational practices, decision-making philosophies, care philosophies, and care work organization (for example, some sources for this information may include pamphlets/brochures, manuals produced for staff or visitors, documents produced by residents'/family members' councils, etc.)

These materials were compiled to form detailed portraits of each LTRC home, its staff (e.g., staff types/mix, staffing levels, shift information), its residents (e.g., demographics, length of stay), and other relevant aspects of its daily policies and practices that would help to familiarize team members with the site prior to starting fieldwork at each LTRC home. This background information also helped researchers to develop initial points of inquiry to take up during the site visits.

Additionally, pre-interviews were conducted by senior researchers on the research team with a few key informants at each site prior to the start of fieldwork and the arrival of the full research team. These pre-interviews were typically conducted with management, union representatives, and/or direct care staff of the home, and were designed to identify some preliminary themes and issues among the various types of workers and to build familiarity with the staff about the project and establish rapport with participants. This allowed research team members to focus on particular points of inquiry upon entering the field – for example, paying particular attention to recent changes in the work organization or policies of the home that were revealed in pre-interviews, and what these changes have meant for residents and relatives. These pre-interviews were also used to seek suggestions for people to interview and to ensure both support for and information about the project for everyone in the nursing home.

An additional key feature of rapid ethnography that was incorporated into the methodology of the Re-imagining LTRC project is that it is conducted as a team, and thus can be considered a type of team ethnography. Our site visits always involved two or more researchers working together on each observation shift, with at least twelve researchers on each site per visit. Following the principles of rapid ethnography, an effort was made to involve a mix of researchers who are more and less familiar with the study site in order to bring new perspectives to both observation in the field and analysis of data (Baines and Cunningham 2011). Gathering ethnographic data as a team has numerous benefits, including both verification of observations as well as a broadening of one's own interpretations through sharing and challenging perspectives with team members from diverse social locations, including differences in gender, race, culture, and discipline (Erickson and Stull 1997). To further maximize these benefits of working as a team, the Re-imagining LTRC project modified the features of rapid ethnography to include an element of *site switching*. The "switching" element refers to the rotation of research team members across the sites and jurisdictions involved in the study. All fieldwork teams were composed of a mix of researchers both from the local context and from among Re-imagining

LTRC's international collaborators. This insider/outsider mix allowed for both familiar and fresh eyes in the field. Local team members offered expertise on the particular setting, including the
absolutely essential ability to translate for fellow team members – in
both the cultural and the linguistic sense – what was seen and heard.
Conversely, non-local team members offered their own expertise
and a point of comparison from the perspective of how LTRC works
within their own countries. By switching team members across sites
and jurisdictions, researchers were able to build comparisons between familiar and unfamiliar settings. The plan was to have the
principle investigator (Pat Armstrong) on all sites to ensure some
overall coordination, but logistics around international travel meant
she did not go to Germany. The program administrator also went
to most sites to manage the data collected and to ensure it was
kept confidential.

The on-site fieldwork for each LTRC home in our study generally
took place over the course of one week. A sample site schedule of
a typical fieldwork week is provided in appendix B, outlining the
team's weekly activities and daily observation shifts. Site schedules
were designed with numerous concerns in mind, the first of which
was the timing of our shift changes. For each site, observation shifts
were designed to begin just before the staff hand-off processes
between shifts, starting with the night-to-morning staff change and
carrying through to the last shift change from evening to night staff,
ensuring that hand-off processes could be observed on all three shifts.
This schedule also meant that, with the exception of the first shift of
the day, oncoming researchers were able to be debriefed by those leaving the home, providing some continuity between shifts. Team members assigned to the last observation shift of the day also often stayed
well beyond the scheduled end time of their shift. This was usually to
obtain interviews with workers who were more available during the
night, or to observe nightly work routines on the invitation of staff,
allowing us to gain a sense of what each LTRC home was like at a time
that is typically unseen by relatives or managerial staff. Observation
shifts were designed to include at least one weekday and one weekend
day, based on the assumption that staff, volunteer, and family activity
might vary between weekdays and weekends.

Following the principles of rapid ethnography, site visits were scheduled to allow for a mix of insiders and outsiders in the research setting simultaneously (Baines and Cunningham 2011). Wherever possible, local researchers were paired with international researchers, students were paired with senior academics, and shifts were composed of team members from different disciplinary backgrounds. These teams changed for each site. This schedule allowed team members to enrich their understandings of the setting and to learn from each other's perspectives. To assist in building rapport with our participants, researchers stayed on the same floor throughout each site visit, while varying the timing of the shifts to allow for a better sense of how activities on the floor differed throughout the day. The team usually met with site managers the evening before the visit started in order to make sure we were all known to those in charge. This evening meeting also allowed members to discuss logistics and familiarize themselves with the approach. The middle of the week was devoted to team meetings for reflection on initial findings and to discuss any challenges or concerns that had been encountered in the field. A similar meeting took place at the end of the week to assess promising practices and the need for additional information or interviews. The mid-week break in observation shifts also allowed time for scheduling interviews with key informants identified during observations on the previous days.

Upon entering an LTRC home for a week of fieldwork, team members used three data-gathering techniques: participant observation, semi-structured interviewing, and "photovoice" interviewing methods. Participant observation involves simultaneously witnessing the activities of others in the setting and participating as a part of that setting, which can range from merely being present in the site to actively participating in the events of that site (Schensul, Schensul, and LeCompte 1999). Our team's participant observation included observing care work in the physical spaces of the LTRC home, as well as the social dynamics that unfolded within these spaces between staff, residents, volunteers, managers, and relatives.

Observational data were recorded through field notes, and team members received training on the goals and methods of ethnographic research as well as note-taking skills and strategies prior to the site visits (Emerson, Fretz, and Shaw 2011). Our team entered the field openly as researchers, introducing ourselves to all participants and wearing name tags throughout the duration of each site visit. Since our researcher identities were not hidden from participants, we were able to jot down a great many field notes "in the moment" during our time at each LTRC home. However, in many instances field notes had to be taken in more private settings or after the fact, given the sensitive nature of many of our observations. When observing conflict or emotionally sensitive moments when it would have been highly inappropriate, uncomfortable, or dangerous for our participants (and our project) to make notes in the open, field notes were instead recorded in secluded areas (e.g., in stairwells, break rooms, and bathrooms) or after leaving the site at the end of an observational shift. An observation guide (see appendix C) was prepared to help researchers focus their field-note writing according to the project's broader research questions (Burgess 1982).

Our site visits also involved conducting interviews with a wide array of workers, family, and volunteers, often taking place spontaneously or scheduled for a later date – typically during the mid-week break in our observation shifts. Having more than one researcher scheduled per observation shift meant that observations of the shift could carry on when one researcher left the floor to conduct interviews. Interviews often involved two team members as interviewers, and many interviews were conducted with multiple participants, resulting in a group interview experience. The research team collaboratively developed interview guides consisting of open-ended questions for each type of participant we would encounter in the field (residents, relatives, nurses, assistive personnel, laundry workers, etc.). Guides were designed to be used in a semi-structured interviewing style, meaning that researchers could ask questions outside of the guide and were free to follow up on points of interest as they occurred throughout the interview. All interviews were digitally recorded and professionally transcribed verbatim, and informed consent was obtained from all participants prior to interviewing and recording. They were immediately transferred to a secure site where data could be shared by all researchers.

Finally, to help minimize the barriers to interview participation facing residents with cognitive or physical challenges that could impair verbal communication, we used the interviewing technique of photovoice. This method combines resident-directed photography with follow-up interviews focused on the content of the photos (Dyches et al. 2004). Photovoice allowed residents with communication challenges a means of conveying ideas and experiences that are important to them, and provided us with insights that we would otherwise have potentially missed through observations and conventional interview techniques alone. Residents were asked not to take pictures of other residents or of staff without permission, and all photos were destroyed after the project.

Sample Site Visit Schedule

	Sunday	Monday	Tuesday	Wednesday	Thursday
UNIT 1					
7 AM–1 PM	PhD student (Norway) Academic (Canada)	Sr academic (Canada) Sr academic (Germany)		Sr academic (Germany) Sr academic (Canada)	Sr academic (Canada) Sr academic (US)
1 PM–7 PM	Sr academic (Canada) Sr academic (Germany)	Sr academic (Sweden) St academic (US)	Team meeting and interviews	Sr academic (Canada) Sr academic (Canada)	Sr academic (Canada) PhD student (Norway)
7 PM–12 AM	Sr academic (Canada) Sr academic (US)	Post-doctoral fellow (Norway) Sr academic (Canada)		Sr academic (Canada) PhD student (Norway)	Sr academic (Canada) Sr academic (Germany)
Unit 2					
7 AM–1 PM	PhD student (US) Sr academic (Canada)	Sr academic (Norway) Post-doctoral fellow (Canada)		Sr academic (Norway) Post-doctoral fellow (Canada)	Sr academic (Canada) Sr academic (Canada)
1 PM–7 PM	Post-doctoral fellow (Canada) Sr academic (Norway)	Sr academic (Canada) Sr academic (Canada)		Sr academic (UK) Sr academic (Canada)	Sr academic (Canada) PhD student (US)
7 PM–12 AM	Sr academic (Canada) Sr academic (Canada)	PhD student (US) Sr academic (Canada)		Sr academic (Canada) PhD student (US)	Post-doctoral fellow (Canada) Sr academic (Norway)

Observation Guide

The following guide was prepared by team members with prior experience in ethnographic methodology. It was provided to the entire research team at the start of each site visit.

Our foci: Active, healthy aging; dignity and respect for residents and staff; processes, practices, and conditions rather than individuals.

Remember that observation is not just watching. Use all senses! Smell, noise, screaming, music, small talk, etc.

- Is the ward calm or chaotic? Are staff rushed? Rushing?
- Describe the physical space. How is it furnished and decorated? Are semipublic spaces decorated by staff? How do they interpret the taste of older people? (bric-a-brac?)
- Describe the spaces for social gatherings, physical layout, accessibility.
- Describe "viewpoints" for people who are too tired to participate (outlook, in busy spaces).
- Think mental, social, and physical stimulation. What works? Does not?
- How are outdoor spaces? How are they used?
- How are residents dressed, based on what? Do they have diapers?

Try to capture the rules, routines, and rhythm of the place. Do residents have a common daily rhythm or do they have their own –

for instance do they eat breakfast alone or with other residents, do
they decide themselves when to get up in the morning and go to
bed in the evening? Can they walk at night? Toileting?

- Is the activity of the place isolated from the community outside
  (people coming in/people going out)?
- How clear are the borders between different spaces? How are
  residents greeted by staff, in what spaces? Do the nurses knock
  before entering the residents' rooms?
- How many staff, of what kinds, doing what? Volunteers? Family?

Try to capture different kinds of events/episodes – staff meetings,
lunch breaks, meals for residents, waking up time, newspaper
reading, physical training, special arrangements (movies, concerts,
picnics, etc.).

Talk to different categories of people and observe how they interact.

- What are the relations between different categories of people,
  e.g. between newcomers and oldtimers, leaders and staff, staff,
  family, volunteers, residents?
- How do leaders provide inspiration, intellectual stimulation, etc.?
- Do family members and guests move freely about the place?
- What kinds of interactions are there between staff members –
  gossip, humour, collegiality, etc.?
- Who is asked and how are they asked to go to social arrangements?

Be aware of your own role and how you are welcomed, how
different people react to you and treat you, and on what basis they
treat you the way they do. Some can see you as outsiders who are
there to judge them or who might have the rhetorical power to
voice their concerns to other outsiders; others may mistake you for a
family member or staff. Take notes discreetly, or remove yourself to
a private space to write them. Do not enter private spaces without
specific consent. Record as much as possible in your notes. No detail
is too small.

ASK YOURSELF WHAT IS MISSING

References

Andrews, John. 2009. "Getting in the Groove." *McKnight's Long-Term Care News*. 1 August. Accessed 29 February 2016. http://www.mcknights.com /news/getting-in-the-groove-making-the-most-out-of-your-laundry-and-housekeeping-team/article/141338/.

– 2011. "Laundry Duty Hazards." *McKnight's Long-Term Care News*. 2 August. Accessed 29 February 2016.http://www.mcknights.com/news/laundry-duty-hazards/article/208396/.

– 2013. "Guardians of Safety." *McKnight's Long-Term Care News*. 1 August. Accessed 29 February 2016. http://www.mcknights.com/news/guardians-of-safety/article/306137/.

Annison, John E. 2000. "Towards a Clearer Understanding of the Meaning of 'Home.'" *Journal of Intellectual and Developmental Disability* 25 (4): 251–62.

Armstrong, Pat. 2013. "Puzzling Skills: Feminist Political Economy Approaches." "50th Anniversary of the *Canadian Review of Sociology*," special issue, *Canadian Review of Sociology* 50 (3): 256–83.

Armstrong, Pat, and Hugh Armstrong. 1978. *The Double Ghetto: Canadian Women and Their Segregated Work*. Toronto: McClelland and Stewart.

– 2004. "Thinking It Through: Women, Work and Caring in the New Millennium." In *Caring For/Caring About: Women, Home Care and Unpaid Caregiving*, edited by Karen R. Grant, Carol Amaratunga, Pat Armstrong, Madeline Boscoe, Ann Pederson, and Kay Willson, 5–44. Aurora: Garamond.

– 2005. "Public and Private: Implications for Care Work." *Sociological Review* 53 (2): 167–87.

– 2009. "Contradictions at Work: Struggles for Control in Canadian Health

Care." In *Morbid Symptoms: Health under Capitalism*, edited by Leo Panitch and Colin Leys, 145–67. Wales: Merlin Press; New York: Monthly Review Press.

– 2010. *Wasting Away: The Undermining of Canadian Health Care*, 2nd edition. Don Mills: Oxford University Press Canada.

– 2016. *About Canada: Health Care*, 2nd edition. Halifax: Fernwood.

Armstrong, Pat, Hugh Armstrong, Albert Banerjee, Tamara Daly, and Marta Szebehely. 2011. "Structural Violence in Long-Term Residential Care." *Women's Health and Urban Life* 10 (1): 111–29.

Armstrong, Pat, Hugh Armstrong, and Krystal Kehoe MacLeod. 2015. "The Threats of Privatization to Security in Long-Term Residential Care." *Ageing International* 41(1): 99-116.

Armstrong, Pat, Hugh Armstrong, and Krista Scott-Dixon. 2008. *Critical to Care: The Invisible Women in Health Services*. Toronto: University of Toronto Press.

Armstrong, Pat, Albert Banerjee, Marta Szebehely, Hugh Armstrong, Tamara Daly, and Stirling Lafrance. 2009. *They Deserve Better: The Long-Term Care Experience in Canada and Scandinavia*. Ottawa: Canadian Centre for Policy Alternatives.

Armstrong, Pat, and Irene Jansen. 2000. "Assessing the Impact of Restructuring and Work Reorganization in Long-Term Care." *National Network on Environments and Women's Health*. Accessed 23 August 2015. http://www.nnewh.org/images/upload/attach/1167armstrong et al 2000.pdf.

Armstrong, Pat, and Olga Kitts. 2004. "One Hundred Years of Caregiving." In *Caring For/Caring About: Women, Home Care and Unpaid Caregiving*, edited by Karen R. Grant, Carol Amaratunga, Pat Armstrong, Madeline Boscoe, Ann Pederson, and Kay Willson, 45–74. Aurora: Garamond.

Armstrong, Pat, and Kate Laxer. 2012. "Demanding Labour: An Aging Health Care Labour Force." Paper presented at the Research Committee (RC) 19 Annual Conference, Oslo, Norway, 25 August.

Armstrong, Pat, and Linda Silas. 2014. "Nurses Unions: Where Knowledge Meets Know-How." In *Realities of Canadian Nursing: Professional, Practice and Power Issues*, edited by Marjorie McIntyre and Carol McDonald, 158–80. New York: Walters Kluwer/Lippincott Williams and Wilkins.

Aronson, Jane, and Sheila M. Neysmith. 1996. "You're Not Just in There to Do the Work: Depersonalizing Policies and the Exploitation of Home Care Workers' Labor." *Gender & Society* 10 (1): 59–77.

Auestad, Reiko Abe. 2010. "Long-Term Care Insurance, Marketization and the Quality of Care: 'Good Time Living' in a Recently Established Nursing Home in a Suburb of Tokyo." *Japan Forum* 21 (2): 209–31.

Austin, Wendy, Erika Goble, Vicki Strang, Agnes Mitchell, Erika Thompson, Helen Lant, Linda Bal, Gillian Lemermeyer, and Kelly Vass. 2009. "Supporting Relationships between Family and Staff in Continuing Care Settings." *Journal of Family Nursing* 15 (3): 360–83.

Baines, Donna. 2004. "Caring for Nothing: Work Organization and Unwaged Labour in Social Services." *Work, Employment and Society* 18(2): 267–95.

– 2006. "Staying with People Who Slap Us Around: Gender, Juggling Responsibilities and Violence in Paid (and Unpaid) Care Work." *Gender, Work and Organization* 13 (2): 129–51.

Baines, Donna, and Pat Armstrong, eds. 2015/2016. *Promising Practices in Long Term Care: Ideas Worth Sharing.* Canadian Centre for Policy Alternatives.

Baines, Donna, and Ian Cunningham. 2011. "Using Comparative Perspective Rapid Ethnography in International Case Studies: Strengths and Considerations." *Qualitative Social Work* 12:73–88.

Balm, Michelle N.D., Roland Jureen, Catherine Teo, Allen E.J. Yeoh, R.T.P. Lin, Stephanie J. Dancer, and D.A. Fisher. 2012. "Hot and Steamy: Outbreak of *Bacillus cereus* in Singapore Associated with Construction Work and Laundry Practices." *Journal of Hospital Infection* 81 (4): 224–30.

Banerjee, Albert. 2010. "On the Frontlines: Structural Violence in Canadian Residential Long-Term Care." PhD diss., York University.

Banerjee, Albert, and Pat Armstrong. 2015. "Centering Care: Explaining Regulatory Tensions in Residential Care for Older Persons." *Studies in Political Economy* 95:7–28.

Banerjee, Albert, Tamara Daly, Hugh Armstrong, Pat Armstrong, Stirling LaFrance, and Marta Szebehely. 2008. *Out of Control: Violence against Personal Support Workers in Long-Term Care.* Toronto: York University.

Banerjee, Albert, Tamara Daly, Pat Armstrong, Marta Szebehely, Hugh Armstrong, and Sterling Lafrance. 2012. "Structural Violence in Long-Term Residential Care for Older People: Comparing Canada and Scandinavia." *Social Science & Medicine* 74 (3): 390–8. doi:10.1016/j.socscimed .2011.10.037.

Bannerji, Himani. 1995. *Thinking Through: Essays on Feminism, Marxism and Anti-Racism.* Toronto: Women's Press.

Barrie, D. 1994. "How Hospital Linen and Laundry Services Are Provided." *Journal of Hospital Infection* 27 (3): 219–35.

Barrie, D., P.N. Hoffman, J.A. Wilson, and J.M. Kramer. 1994. "Contamination of Hospital Linen by *Bacillus cereus*." *Epidemiology and Infection* 113 (2): 297–306.

Bayer, Tony, Win Tadd, and Stefan Krajcik. 2005. "Dignity: The Voice of Older People." *Quality in Ageing and Older Adults* 6 (1): 22–9.

Beechey, Veronica. 1982. "The Sexual Division of Labour and the Labour Process: A Critical Assessment of Braverman." In *The Degradation of Work? Skill, Deskilling and the Labour Process*, edited by Stephen Wood, 54–73. London: Hutchinson.

Bergland, Ådel. 2005. "Resident–Caregiver Relationships and Thriving among Nursing Home Residents." *Research in Nursing & Health* 28 (5): 365–75.

Berta, Whitney, Audrey Laporte, and Walter P. Wodchis. 2014. "Approaches to Accountability in Long-Term Care." *Healthcare Policy* 10 (SP): 132–44.

Bland, Marian. 2005. "The Challenge of Feeling 'At Home' in Residential Aged Care in New Zealand." *Nursing Praxis in New Zealand* 21:4–12.

– 2007. "Betwixt and Between: A Critical Ethnography of Comfort in New Zealand Residential Aged Care." *Journal of Clinical Nursing* 16:937–44.

Borg, Michael, and A. Portelli. 1999. "Hospital Laundry Workers: An At-Risk Group for Hepatitis A?" *Occupational Medicine* 49 (7): 448–50.

Borrie, Michael, and Heather A. Davidson. 1992. "Incontinence in Institutions: Costs and Contributing Factors." *Canadian Medical Association Journal* 147 (3): 322–8.

Bowblis, John, and Kathryn Hyer. 2013. "Nursing Home Staffing Requirements and Input Substitution: Effects on Housekeeping, Food Service, and Activities Staff." *Health Services Research* 48 (4): 1539–50.

Bowers, Barbara, Kim Nolet, Tonya Roberts, and Sarah Esmond. 2009. *Implementing Change in Long-Term Care: A Practical Guide to Transformation*. New York: The Commonwealth Fund.

Braverman, Harry. 1974. *Labor and Monopoly Capital: The Degradation of Work in the Twentieth Century*. New York: Monthly Review Press.

Buchanan, Dan. 2011. "The Not-for-Profit Contribution and Issues from the Provider Perspective." Paper presented at Reimagining Long-Term Residential Care Annual Meeting, Toronto, 2 June.

Burgess, Robert G. 1982. *Field Research: A Sourcebook and Manual*. London, UK: George Allen and Unwin.

Buse, Christina, and Julia Twigg. 2014. "Looking 'Out of Place': Analysing the Spatial and Symbolic Meanings of Dementia Care Settings through Dress." *International Journal of Ageing and Later Life* 9 (1): 69–95.

– 2015. "Clothing, Embodied Identity and Dementia: Maintaining the Self through Dress." *Age, Culture, Humanities* 2:1–31.

– 2016. "Materialising Memories: Exploring the Stories of People with Dementia through Dress." *Ageing and Society* 36 (6): 1115–35.

Butler, Judith. 1990. *Gender Trouble and the Subversion of Identity.* New York: Routledge.

Calnan, Michael, David Badcott, and Gillian Woolhead. 2006. "Dignity under Threat? A Study of the Experiences of Older People in the United Kingdom." *International Journal of Health Services* 36 (2): 355–75. doi:10.2190/0DJ2-JE0X-X2HR-EU7E.

Campbell, Andrea. 2013. "Work Organization, Care, and Occupational Health and Safety." In *Troubling Care: Critical Perspectives on Research and Practices,* edited by Pat Armstrong and Susan Braedley, 89–100. Toronto: Canadian Scholars' Press Inc.

Canadian Healthcare Association. 2009. *New Directions for Facility-Based Long-Term Care.* Ottawa: Canadian Healthcare Association.

Canadian Union of Public Employees (CUPE). 2003. "Laundry Service Workers: Critical to Care." *CUPE.ca.* Accessed 14 September 2015. http://archive .cupe.ca/updir/Laundryrev.pdf.

– 2009. "Healthcare Associated Infections: A Backgrounder." *CUPE.ca.* Accessed 15 September 2015. http://cupe.ca/health-care-associated-infections-backgrounder-and-fact-sheet.

– 2013. "Backgrounder on K-Bro Linen Systems: The New Provider of Hospital Linens in Saskatchewan." *CUPE.ca.* Accessed 16 March 2015. http://sk.cupe.ca/files/2013/04/Final-K-Bro-Backgrounder-_CUPE_December-17-2013.pdf.

Castle, Nicholas G. 2007. "A Review of Satisfaction Instruments Used in Long-Term Care Settings." *Journal of Aging and Social Policy* 19 (2): 9–41.

– 2008. "Nursing Home Caregiver Staffing Levels and Quality of Care: A Literature Review." *Journal of Applied Gerontology* 27:375–405. doi:10.1177/0733464808321596.

Castle, Nicholas, and Fran Sheedy Bost. 2009. "Perfecting Patient Care: Integrating Principles of Process Redesign in Nursing Homes." *Journal of Applied Gerontology* 28 (2): 256–76.

Charras, Kevin, and Fabrice Gzil. 2013. "Judging a Book by Its Cover: Uniforms and Quality of Life in Special Care Units for People with Dementia." *American Journal of Alzheimer's Disease and Other Dementias* 28 (5): 450–8.

Chau, Janita P., David R. Thompson, D.T. Lee, and Sheila Twinn. 2010. "Infection Control Practices among Hospital Health and Support Workers in Hong Kong." *Journal of Hospital Infection* 75 (4): 299–303.

Choiniere, Jacqueline, Malcolm Doupe, Monika Goldmann, Frode Jacobsen, Liz Lloyd, Magali Rootham, and Marta Szebehely. 2016. "Mapping Nursing Home Inspections and Audits in Six Countries." *Ageing International* 41 (1): 40–61.

Chowdhary, Usha. 1991. "Clothing and Self-Esteem of the Institutionalized Elderly Female: Two Experiments." *Educational Gerontology* 17 (6): 527–41.

Cohen, Marcy. 2006. "The Privatization of Health Care Cleaning Services in Southwestern British Columbia, Canada: Union Responses to Unprecedented Government Action." *Antipode* 38 (3): 626–44.

Cohen, Marjorie Griffin. 2001. "Do Comparisons between Hospital Support Workers and Hospitality Workers Make Sense?" *Hospital Employees' Union.* Accessed 15 August 2015. http://www.heu.org/sites/default /files/uploads/research_reports/Comparison_Hospital_Support_Workers _1.pdf.

Cohen, Marjorie Griffin, and Marcy Cohen. 2004. "A Return to Wage Discrimination: Pay Equity Losses through the Privatization of Health Care." *Canadian Centre for Policy Alternatives.* Accessed 19 March 2015. http://www.policyalternatives.ca/sites/default/files/uploads/publications /BC_Office_Pubs/bc_pay_equity.pdf.

Connelly, M. Patricia, and Pat Armstrong, eds. 1992. *Feminism in Action: Studies in Political Economy.* Toronto: Canadian Scholars Press.

Coyle, Angela. 2005. "Changing Times: Flexibilization and the Re-organization of Work in Feminized Labour Markets." *Sociological Review* 53 (S2): 73–88.

Cummings, Valerie, Rhonda Holt, Carolin van der Sloot, Katherine Moore, and Derek Griffiths. 1995. "Costs and Management of Urinary Incontinence in Long-Term Care." *Journal of Wound, Ostomy, and Continence Nursing* 22 (4): 193–8.

Daly, Tamara. 2015. "Dancing the Two-Step in Ontario's Long-Term Care Sector: Deterrence Regulation = Consolidation." *Studies in Political Economy* 95:29–58.

Daly, Tamara, Pat Armstrong, and Ruth Lowndes. 2015. "Liminality in Ontario's Long-Term Care Facilities: Private Companions' Care Work in the Space 'Betwixt and Between.'" *Competition & Change* 3 (19): 246–63.

Daly, Tamara, Albert Banerjee, Pat Armstrong, Hugh Armstrong, and Marta Szebehely. 2011. "Lifting the 'Violence Veil': Examining Working Conditions in Long-Term Care Facilities Using Iterative Mixed Methods." *Canadian Journal on Aging* 30 (2): 271–84.

Daly, Tamara, and Marta Szebehely. 2012. "Unheard Voices, Unmapped Terrain: Care Work in Long-Term Residential Care for Older People in Canada and Sweden." *International Journal of Social Welfare* 21 (2): 139–48.

Dancer, Stephanie J. 2009. "The Role of Environmental Cleaning in the Control of Hospital-Acquired Infection." *Journal of Hospital Infection* 73 (4): 378–85.

– 2011. "Hospital Cleaning in the 21st Century." *European Journal of Clinical Microbiology and Infectious Diseases* 30 (12): 1473–81.

Das Gupta, Tania, Rebecca Hagey, and Jane Turritin. 2007. "Racial Discrimination in Nursing." In *Interrogating Race and Racism*, edited by Vijay Agnew, 261–301. Toronto: University of Toronto Press.

Day, Suzanne. 2013. "The Implications of Conceptualizing Care." In *Troubling Care: Critical Perspectives on Research and Practices*, edited by Pat Armstrong and Susan Braedley, 21–32. Toronto: Canadian Scholars' Press.

– 2014. "Making It Work: A Study of the Decision-Making Processes of Personal Support Workers in Long-Term Residential Care." PhD diss., York University.

DeForge, Ryan, Paul Van Wyk, Jodi Catherine Hall, and Alan Salmoni. 2011. "Afraid to Care, Unable to Care: A Critical Ethnography within a Long-Term Care Home." *Journal of Aging Studies* 25 (4): 415–26.

Dempsey, Nora P., and Rachel A. Pruchno. 1993. "The Family's Role in the Nursing Home: Predictors of Technical and Non-Technical Assistance." *Journal of Gerontological Social Work* 21 (1–2): 127–46.

Denton, Margaret, Catherine Brookman, Isik Zeytinoglu, Jennifer Plenderleith, and Rachel Barken. 2014. "Task Shifting in the Provision of Home and Social Care in Ontario, Canada: Implications for Quality of Care." *Health & Social Care in the Community* 23 (5): 485–92. doi:10.1111 /hsc.12168.

Denton, Miles, M.H. Wilcox, Peter Parnell, D. Green, V. Keer, P.M. Hawkey, I. Evans, and P. Murphy. 2004. "Role of Environmental Cleaning in Controlling an Outbreak of *Acinetobacter baumannii* on a Neurosurgical Intensive Care Unit." *Journal of Hospital Infection* 56 (2): 106–10.

Diamond, Timothy. 1986. "Social Policy and Everyday Life in Nursing Homes: A Critical Ethnography." *Social Science and Medicine* 23:1287–95.

– 1992. *Making Gray Gold: Narratives of Nursing Home Care*. Chicago, Illinois: University of Chicago Press.

Dobbs, Debra J., Kevin Eckert, Bob Rubinstein, Lynn Keimig, Leanne Clark, Ann Christine Frankowski, and Sheryl Zimmerman. 2008. "An Ethnographic Study of Stigma and Ageism in Residential Care or Assisted Living." *Gerontologist* 48 (4): 517–26.

Dodson, Lisa, and Rebekah M. Zincavage. 2007. "'It's Like a Family': Caring Labor, Exploitation, and Race in Nursing Homes." *Gender & Society* 21(6): 905–28.

Donaldson, Tria, and Cheryl Stadnichuk. 2015. "Lessons from Laundry Privatization: Why Freedom of Information Matters in the Era of Privatization." *Rankandfile.ca: Canadian Labour News Website*. Accessed 15 August 2015. http://rankandfile.ca/2015/08/05/lessons-from-laundry-privatization-why-freedom-of-information-matters-in-the-era-of-privatization/.

Dryden, Robert, and Jim Stanford. 2012. *The Unintended Consequences of Outsourcing Cleaning Work*. Ottawa: Canadian Centre for Policy Alternatives.

Duckett, Stephen. 2012. *Where to from Here? Keeping Medicare Sustainable*. Montreal and Kingston: McGill-Queen's University Press.

Duffy, Jonathan, Julie Harris, Lilitha Gade, Lynne Sehulster, Emily Newhouse, Heather O'Connell, Judith Noble-Wang, Carol Rao, S.A. Balajee, and Tom Chiller. 2014. "Mucormycosis Outbreak Associated with Hospital Linens." *Pediatric Infectious Disease Journal* 33 (5): 472–6. doi:10.1097 /INF.0000000000000261.

Dyches, Tina Taylor, Elizabeth Cichella, Susanne Frost Olsen, and Barbara Mandleco. 2004. "Snapshots of Life: Perspectives of School-Aged Individuals with Developmental Disabilities." *Research and Practices for Persons with Severe Disabilities* 29:172–82.

Dyck, Isabel, Pia Kontos, Jan Angus, and Patricia McKeever. 2005. "The Home as a Site for Long-Term Care: Meanings and Management of Bodies and Spaces." *Health & Place* 11 (2): 173–85.

Eckenwiler, Lisa A. 2012. *Long-Term Care, Globalization and Justice*. Baltimore: The Johns Hopkins University Press.

Egan, Kelly. 1997a. "Cobden Nursing Home to Close: 'Devastated' Seniors May Be Forced to Leave Village." *Ottawa Citizen*, 10 July.

– 1997b. "Heartbroken in Cobden: Many Are 'Wounded in the Mind', but Residents of Lakeview Nursing Home Are Part of Community's Fabric." *Ottawa Citizen*, 11 September.

Ejaz, Farida K., Linda S. Noelker, Dorothy Schur, Carol J. Whitlatch, and Wendy J. Looman. 2002. "Family Satisfaction with Nursing Home Care for Relatives with Dementia." *Journal of Applied Gerontology* 21 (3): 368–84.

Emerson, Robert M., Rachel I. Fretz, and Linda L. Shaw. 2011. *Writing Ethnographic Fieldnotes*. Chicago, Illinois: University of Chicago Press.

Entwistle, Joanne. 2001. "The Dressed Body." In *Body Dressing: Dress, Body, Culture*, edited by Joanne Enwistle and Elizabeth Wilson, 33–58. Oxford: Berg.

Erickson, Ken C., and Donald D. Stull. 1997. *Doing Team Ethnography: Warnings and Advice*. Thousand Oaks, California: Sage Publications.

Erlandson, Sara, Palle Storm, Anneli Stranz, Marta Szebehely, and Gun-Britt Trydegård. 2013. "Marketization Trends in Swedish Eldercare: Competition, Choice and Calls for Stricter Regulation." In *Marketization in Nordic Eldercare: A Research Report on Legislation, Oversight, Extent and Consequences*, edited by Gabrielle Meagher and Marta Szebehely, 23–83. Stockholm: Stockholm University.

Esping-Andersen, Gosta. 1990. *The Three Worlds of Welfare Capitalism*. Princeton, NJ: Princeton University Press.

European Agency for Safety and Health at Work. 2003. *Gender Issues in Safety and Health at Work: A Review*. Luxembourg: European Union.

Evans, Robert G. 1997. "Going for the Gold: The Redistributive Agenda behind Market-Based Health Care Reform." *Journal of Health Politics, Policy and Law* 22 (2): 427–65.

Ferrie, Jane E., Martin J. Shipley, Katherine Newman, Stephen A. Stansfeld, and Michael G. Marmot. 2005. "Self-Reported Job Insecurity and Health in the Whitehall II Study: Potential Explanations of the Relationship." *Social Science and Medicine* 60 (7): 1593–602.

Fijan, Sabina, and Sonja Sostar-Turk. 2012. "Hospital Textiles, Are They a Possible Vehicle for Healthcare-Associated Infections?" *International Journal of Environmental Research and Public Health* 9 (9): 3330–43.

Fijan, Sabina, Sonja Sostar-Turk, and Avrelija Cencic. 2005. "Implementing Hygiene Monitoring Systems in Hospital Laundries in Order to Reduce

Microbial Contamination of Hospital Textiles." *Journal of Hospital Infection Control* 61 (1): 30–8.

Fine, Michael. 2007. "The Social Division of Care." *The Australian Journal of Social Issues* 42 (2): 137–49.

Foner, Nancy. 1994. *The Caregiving Dilemma: Work in an American Nursing Home*. Berkley, CA: University of California Press.

Forastieri, Valentina. 2000. "Important Note on Women Workers and Gender Issues on Occupational Safety and Health." *International Programme on Safety Health and the Environment*. Geneva: ILO Safe Work.

Friedman, Milton. 1962. *Capitalism and Freedom*. Chicago: University of Chicago Press.

Galvin, Kathleen, and Les Todres. 2013. *Caring and Well-Being: A Lifeworld Approach*. Oxfordshire: Routledge.

Gaubert, Nathan S. 2010. "Proper Laundry Protocol." *Long-Term Living* 59 (1): 32–3.

Glenn, Evelyn Nakano. 2010. *Forced to Care: Coercion and Caregiving in America*. Cambridge: Harvard University Press.

Goodsell, Devon. 2012. "B.C.'s Privatization of Seniors' Care Raises Concerns." *CBC News*. Accessed 8 May 2015. http://www.cbc.ca/news/canada /british-columbia/story/2012/05/07/bc-seniors-business-private.html.

Goodwin, S. 1994. "Personal Laundry: An Essential Part of Patient Care." *Nursing Times* 90 (30): 31–2.

Government of Canada. 1984. "Canada Health Act." *Government of Canada Justice Laws*. Accessed 29 February 2016. http://laws-lois.justice.gc.ca/eng /acts/C-6/FullText.html.

Government of New Brunswick. 2013. "Further Savings to Be Achieved by Nursing Homes Sharing Laundry Services." *Government of New Brunswick*. Accessed 10 April 2015. http://www2.gnb.ca/content/gnb/en/news/news _release.2013.02.0150.html.

Government of the United Kingdom. 2015. "Contract Types and Employer Responsibilities." *Government of the United Kingdom*. Accessed 29 February 2016. https://www.gov.uk/contract-types-and-employer-responsibilities /zero-hour-contracts.

Grant, Hugh, Manish Pandey, and James Townsend. 2014. "Short-Term Gain, Long-Term Pain: The Privatization of Hospital Laundry Services in Saskatchewan." *Canadian Centre for Policy Alternatives*. Accessed 19 April 2015. https://www.policyalternatives.ca/sites/default/files/uploads

/publications/Saskatchewan Office/2015/01/SK_Privatization_of
_Hospital_Laundry.pdf.

Grant, Karen R., Carol Amaratunga, Pat Armstrong, Madeline Boscoe, Ann
Pederson, and Kay Willson, eds. 2004. *Caring For/Caring About: Women,
Home Care and Unpaid Caregiving.* Aurora: Garamond Press.

Greig, Judy, and M.B. Lee. 2009. "Enteric Outbreaks in Long-Term Care
Facilities and Recommendations for Prevention: A Review." *Epidemiology
and Infection* 137 (3): 145–55.

Gubrium, Jaber F. 1975. *Living and Dying at Murray Manor.* Charlotteville,
VA: University Press of Virginia.

Gunnarsdóttir, S., and K. Björnsdóttir. 2003. "Health Promotion in the
Workplace: The Perspective of Unskilled Workers in a Hospital Setting."
Scandinavian Journal of Caring Sciences 17 (1): 66–73.

Habjanic, Ana, and Majda Pajnkihar. 2013. "Family Members' Involvement
in Elder Care Provision in Nursing Homes and Their Considerations
about Financial Compensation: A Qualitative Study." *Archives of Gerontology and Geriatrics* 56 (3): 425–31.

Hall, Ellen M. 1992. "Double Exposure: The Combined Impact of the Home
and Work Environments on Psychosomatic Strain in Swedish Women and
Men." *International Journal of Health Services* 22 (2): 239–60.

Hallgrimsdottir, Helga K., Katherine Teghtsoonian, and Debra Brown. 2008.
"Public Policy, Caring Practices and Gender in Health Care Work." *Canadian Journal of Public Health* 99 (2): 43–7.

Handwerker, W. Pen. 2001. *Quick Ethnography.* Walnut Creek, CA: Altamira
Press.

Hannah-Moffat, Kelly, and Pat O'Malley. 2007. *Gendered Risks.* New York:
Routledge.

Harbers, Hans, Annemarie Mol, and Alice Stollmeyer. 2002. "Food Matters:
Arguments for an Ethnography of Daily Care." *Theory, Culture and Society*
19:207–26.

Harnett, Tove. 2010. "Seeking Exemptions from Nursing Home Routines:
Residents' Everyday Influence Attempts and Institutional Order." *Journal
of Aging Studies* 24(4): 292–301.

Harrington, Charlene. 2013. "Understanding the Relationship of Nursing
Home Ownership and Quality in the United States." In *Marketization in
Nordic Eldercare: A Research Report on Legislation, Oversight, Extent and
Consequences,* edited by Gabrielle Meagher and Marta Szebehely, 229–40.
Stockholm: Stockholm University.

Harrington, Charlene, Hugh Armstrong, Mark Halladay, Anders Kvale Havig, Frode Jacobsen, Martha MacDonald, Justin Panos, Kathy Pearsall, Allyson Pollock, and Leslie Ross. 2016. "Comparison of Nursing Home Financial Transparency and Accountability in Four Locations." *Ageing International* 41 (1): 17–39.

Harrington, Charlene, Jacqueline Choiniere, Monika Goldmann, Frode Fadnes Jacobsen, Liz Lloyd, Margaret McGregor, Vivian Stamatopoulos, and Marta Szebehely. 2012. "Nursing Home Staffing Standards and Staffing Levels in Six Countries." *The Journal of Nursing Scholarship* 44 (1): 88–98.

Harrington, Charlene, Brian Olney, Helen Carrillo, and Taewoon Kang. 2012. "Nurse Staffing and Deficiencies in the Largest For-Profit Nursing Home Chains and Chains Owned by Private Equity Companies." *Health Services Research* 47 (1): 106–28.

Hayek, Friedrich A. 1944. *The Road to Serfdom*. Chicago: University of Chicago Press.

Hsu, Amy T., Whitney Berta, Peter C. Coyte, and Audrey Laporte. 2016. "Staffing in Ontario's Long-Term Care Homes: Differences in Profit Status and Chain Ownership." *Canadian Journal on Ageing* 35 (2): 175–89.

Hu, Tei, D. Kaltreider, and Jessie F. Iguo. 1990. "The Cost Effectiveness of Disposable versus Reusable Diapers: A Controlled Experiment in a Nursing Home." *Gerontological Nursing* 16 (2): 19–24.

Hynd, Tamara. 2015. "Interior Health Closer to Privatizing Laundry Services in Nelson." *Nelson Star*, 11 February.

Jacobsen, Frode F., and Tone Elin Mekki. 2012. "Health and the Changing Welfare State in Norway: A Focus on Municipal Health Care for Elderly Sick." *Ageing International* 37:125–42.

Kamp, Annette, and Helge Hvid. 2012. "Introduction: Elderly Care in Transition." In *Elderly Care in Transition: Management, Meaning and Identity at Work: A Scandinavian Perspective*, edited by Annette Kamp and Helge Hvid, 13–28. Copenhagen: Copenhagen Business School Press.

Kapucu, Naim. 2006. "New Public Management: Theory, Ideology and Practice." In *Handbook of Globalization, Governance, and Public Administration*, edited by Ali Farazmand and Jack Pinkowski, 885–9. Boca Raton: Taylor and Francis.

Karasek, Robert A. 1979. "Job Demands, Job Decision Latitude, and Mental Strain: Implications for Job Redesign." *Administrative Science Quarterly* 24 (2): 285–308.

Keefe, Janice, and Pamela Fancey. 2000. "The Care Continues: Responsibility for Elderly Relatives before and after Admission to a Long Term Care Facility." *Family Relations* 49 (3): 235–44.

Knijn, Trudie, and Monique Kremer. 1997. "Gender and the Caring Dimension of Welfare States: Towards Inclusive Citizenship." *Social Politics* 4 (3): 328–61.

Kofman, Eleonore, and Parvati Raghuram. 2006. "Gender and Global Labour Migrations: Incorporating Skilled Workers." *Antipode* 38 (2): 282–303.

Kontos, Pia C. 2004. "Ethnographic Reflections on Selfhood, Embodiment and Alzheimer's Disease." *Ageing and Society* 24 (6): 829–49.

Kontos, Pia C., Karen-Lee Miller, and Gail J. Mitchell. 2010. "Neglecting the Importance of the Decision Making and Care Regimes of Personal Support Workers: A Critique of Standardization of Care Planning through RAI/MDS." *The Gerontologist* 50 (3): 352–62.

Kovacs, Steve. 2012. "Laundry and Long Term Care: Providers Can Improve the Bottom Line and Boost Customer Satisfaction with Some Everyday Laundry Essentials." *Provider Magazine*, 1 February. Accessed 25 February 2015. http://www.providermagazine.com/archives/archives-2012/Pages /0212/Laundry-And-Long-Term-Care.aspx.

Kumar, M. Shashi, B. Ramakrishna Goud, and Bobby Joseph. 2014. "A Study of the Occupational Health and Safety Measures in the Laundry Department of a Private Tertiary Care Teaching Hospital, Bengaluru." *Indian Journal of Occupational and Environmental Medicine* 18 (1): 13–20.

Lászlóa, Krisztina D., Hynek Pikhartc, Maria S. Koppa, Martin Bobakc, Andrzej Pajakd, Sofia Malyutinae, Gyöngyvér Salavecza, and Michael Marmotc. 2010. "Job Insecurity and Health: A Study of 16 European Countries." *Social Science and Medicine* 70 (6): 867–74.

Laxer, Katherine. 2015. "Who Counts in Care? Gender, Power, and Aging Populations." In *Women's Health: Intersections of Policy, Research, and Practice*, edited by Pat Armstrong and Ann Pederson, 212–37. Toronto: Women's Press.

– 2013. "Counting Carers in Long-Term Residential Care in Canada." In *Troubling Care: Critical Perspectives on Research and Practices*, edited by Pat Armstrong and Susan Braedley, 73–88. Toronto: Canadian Scholars' Press.

Laxer, Katherine, Frode F. Jacobsen, Liz Lloyd, Monika Goldmann, Suzanne Day, Jacqueline A. Choiniere, and Pauline Vaillancourt Rosenau. 2016.

"Comparing Nursing Home Assistive Personnel in Five Countries." *Ageing International* 41 (1): 62–78. doi:10.1007/s12126-015-9226-2.

Lee-Treweek, Geraldine. 1997. "Women, Resistance and Care: An Ethnographic Study of Nursing Auxiliary Work." *Work, Employment & Society* 11 (1): 47–63.

Leira, Arnlaug, and Chiara Saraceno. 2002. "Care: Actors, Relationships and Contexts." In *Contested Concepts in Gender and Social Politics*, edited by Barbara Hobson, Jane Lewis, and Birte Siim, 55–83. Cheltenham: Edward Elgar.

Leith, Katherine H. 2006. "Home Is Where the Heart Is ... or Is It? A Phenomenological Exploration of the Meaning of Home for Older Women in Congregate Housing." *Journal of Aging Studies* 20 (4): 317–33.

Lippel, Katherine. 2003. "Compensation for Musculo-Skeletal Disorders in Quebec: Systemic Discrimination against Women Workers?" *International Journal of Health Services* 33 (2): 253–81.

Lloyd, Liz, Albert Banerjee, Charlene Harrington, Frode F. Jacobsen, and Marta Szebehely. 2014. "It Is a Scandal! Comparing the Causes and Consequences of Nursing Home Media Scandals in Five Countries." *International Journal of Sociology and Social Policy* 34 (1/2): 2–18.

Lopez, Stephen H. 2006a. "Culture Change Management in Long-Term Care: A Shop-Floor View." *Politics and Society* 34:55–70.

– 2006b. "Emotional Labor and Organized Emotional Care." *Work and Occupations* 33:133–60.

– 2007. "Efficiency and the Fix Revisited: Informal Relations and Mock Routinization in a Nonprofit Nursing Home." *Qualitative Sociology* 30:225–47.

Louther, Joyce, Pedro Rivera, Joseph Feldman, Noreida Villa, Jack DeHovitz, and K.A. Sepkowitz. 1997. "Risk of Tuberculin Conversion According to Occupation among Health Care Workers at a New York City Hospital." *American Journal of Respiratory and Critical Care Medicine* 156 (1): 201–5.

Luxton, Meg. 1980. *More Than a Labour of Love: Three Generations of Women's Work in the Home*. Toronto: The Canadian Women's Educational Press.

Luxton, Meg, and Kate Bezanson. 2006. *Social Reproduction: Feminist Political Economy Challenges Neo-Liberalism*. Montreal and Kingston: McGill-Queen's University Press.

MacDonald, Martha. 1991. "Post Fordism and the Flexibility Debate." *Studies in Political Economy* 36 (Fall): 177–201.

Maher, L. 2001. "A New Spin on an Old Issue: Airing Solutions about Dirty Laundry." *Contemporary Longterm Care* 24 (11): 20–4.

Marmot, Michael G., Geoffrey Rose, Martin Shipley, and P.J.S. Hamilton. 1978. "Employment Grade and Coronary Heart Disease in British Civil Servants." *Journal of Epidemiology and Community Health* 32 (4): 244–9. doi:10.1136/jech.32.4.244.

Marmot, Michael G., G. Davey Smith, Stephen Stansfield, C. Patel, F. North, J. Head, I. White, E. Brunner, and A. Feeney. 1991. "Health Inequalities among British Civil Servants: The Whitehall II Study." *Lancet* 337 (8754): 1387–93. doi:10.1016/0140-6736(91)93068-K.

Marmot, Michael, and Richard G. Wilkinson. 2006. *Social Determinants of Health*, 2nd ed. New York: Oxford University Press.

McColgan, Gillian. 2005. "A Place to Sit: Resistance Strategies Used to Create Privacy and Home by People with Dementia." *Journal of Contemporary Ethnography* 34:410–33.

McDonough, Peggy. 2000. "Job Insecurity and Health." *International Journal of Health Services* 30 (3): 453–76.

McGilton, Katherine S., Sepali Guruge, Ruby Librado, Lois Bloch, and Veronique Boscart. 2008. "Health Care Aides' Struggle to Build and Maintain Relationships with Families in Complex Continuing Care Settings." *Canadian Journal on Aging* 27 (2): 135–43.

McGregor, Margaret J., Marcy Cohen, Kim McGrail, Anne Marie Broemeling, Reva Adler, Michael Schulzer, Lisa Ronald, Yuri Cvitkovich, and Mary Beck. 2005. "Staffing Levels in Not-for-Profit and For-Profit Long-Term Care Facilities: Does Type of Ownership Matter?" *Canadian Medical Association Journal* 172 (5): 645–9.

McGregor, Margaret J., Marcy Cohen, Catherine-Rose Stocks-Rankin, Michelle B. Cox, Kia Salomons, Kimberlyn M. McGrail, Charmaine Spencer, Lisa A. Ronald, and Michael Schultzer. 2011. "Complaints in For-Profit, Non-Profit and Public Nursing Homes in Two Canadian Provinces." *Open Medicine* 5 (4): e183–92.

McGregor, Margaret J., and Lisa A. Ronald. 2011. *Residential Long-Term Care for Canadian Seniors: Nonprofit, For-Profit or Does It Matter?* Montreal: Institute for Research on Public Policy.

McKay, Paul. 2003a. "The Missing Millions of a Nursing Home Empire: Ontario's Nursing Home Crisis – Part 2." *Ottawa Citizen*, 27 April.

– 2003b. "Mining Florida's Seniors for Gold: Ontario's Nursing Home Crisis – Part 3." *Ottawa Citizen*, 28 April.

– 2003c. "Taxpayers Finance Construction Boom: Ontario's Nursing Home Crisis — Part 4." *Ottawa Citizen*, 29 April.

Meagher, Gabrielle, and Marta Szebehely. 2013. *Marketization in Nordic*

Eldercare: A Research Report on Legislation, Oversight, Extent and Consequences. Stockholm: Stockholm University.

Messing, Karen. 1997. "Women's Occupational Health: A Critical Review and Discussion of Current Issues." *Women and Health* 25 (4): 39–68.

– 1998a. *One-Eyed Science: Occupational Health and Women Workers*. Philadelphia: Temple University Press.

– 1998b. "Hospital Trash: Cleaners Speak of Their Role in Disease Prevention." *Medical Anthropology Quarterly* 12 (2): 168–87.

Messing, Karen, Katherine Lippel, Diane L. Demers, and Donna Mergler. 2000. "Equality and Difference in the Workplace: Physical Job Demands, Occupational Illnesses, and Sex Differences." *National Women's Studies Association Journal* 12 (3): 21–49.

Milch, Bernard. 1995. "On-Premises Laundry Equipment: Exploring the Options." *Nursing Homes* 44 (8): 36.

Millen, David R. 2000. "Rapid Ethnography: Time Deepening Strategies for HCI Field Research." Paper presented at DIS '00, the 3rd conference on Designing Interactive Systems: Processes, Practices, Methods, and Techniques. Brooklyn, New York, 17–19 August.

Milmo, Cahal. 2013. "Britain's Cruelest Care Home: 'Institutional Abuse' Contributed to Deaths of Five Pensioners." *Independent*, 18 October. Accessed 29 February 2016. http://www.independent.co.uk/news/uk /home-news/britains-cruellest-care-home-institutional-abuse-contributed- to-deaths-of-five-pensioners-8889770.html.

Moultrie, Keith, Ruth Bartlett, Kim Foo, Lenanne Whitehead, and Neil Duce. 2005. "Mapping the Service User's Journey: A Care Pathway Approach to Raising Standards in Long-Term Care." *Dementia* 4 (3): 442.

Ness, Immanuel, and Roland Zullo. 2003. "Privatization, Labor-Management Relations, and Working Conditions for Lower-Skilled Workers of Color." *Poverty and Race Research Action Council*. Accessed 29 February 2016. http://www.prrac.org/full_text.php?text_id=931&item_id=8336 &newsletter_id=69&header=Employment+%2F+Labor+%2F+Jobs +Policy.

Neysmith, S.M. 1991. "From Community Care to a Social Model of Care." In *Women's Caring: Feminist Perspectives on Social Welfare*, edited by Carol T. Baines, Patricia M. Evans, and Sheila M. Neysmith, 272–99. Toronto: McClelland & Stewart Inc.

Noddings, Nel. 1984. *Caring: A Feminine Approach to Ethics and Moral Education*. Berkley, CA: University of California Press.

Ontario Auditor General. 2015. "Annual Report 2015." *Office of the Auditor General of Ontario*. Accessed 29 February 2016. http://www.auditor.on.ca /en/reports_2015_en.htm.

Ontario Ministry of Health and Long-Term Care. 2008. "Important Changes to LTC Home Compliance." *Ontario Ministry of Health and Long-Term Care Website*. Accessed 22 September 2015. http://www.health.gov.on.ca/en/public/programs/ltc/trans_project.aspx.

Organisation for Economic Co-operation and Development. 2011. "Help Wanted? Providing and Paying for Long-Term Care." *OECD.org*. Accessed 29 February 2016. http://www.oecd.org/els/health-systems/47884930.pdf.

– 2015. "Health at a Glance 2015." *OECD.org*. Accessed 29 February 2016. http://www.keepeek.com/Digital-Asset-Management/oecd/social-issues-migration-health/health-at-a-glance-2015_health_glance-2015-en#.

Oswald, Frank, and Hans-Werner Wahl. 2005. "Dimensions of the Meaning of Home in Later Life." In *Home and Identity in Late Life: International Perspectives*, edited by Graham D. Rowles and Habib Chaudhury, 21–44. New York: Springer.

Power, Michael. 1999. *The Audit Society: Rituals of Verification*. Oxford: Oxford University Press.

Powers, Bethel Ann. 2003. "The Significance of Losing Things: For Nursing Home Residents with Dementia and Their Families." *Journal of Gerontological Nursing* 29 (11): 43–52.

Prada, Gabriella. 2011. *Innovation Procurement in Health Care: A Compelling Opportunity for Canada*. Ottawa: Conference Board of Canada.

Public Health Agency of Canada. 2011. "What Determines Health?" *Public Health Agency of Canada*. Accessed 29 February 2016. http://www.phac-aspc.gc.ca/ph-sp/determinants/index-eng.php.

Public Services International Research Unit. 2014. "Public and Private Sector Efficiency." *A Briefing for the EPSU Congress by PSIRU*. Accessed 29 February 2016. http://www.psiru.org/sites/default/files/2014-07-EWGHT-efficiency.pdf.

Puddephatt, Anthony J., William Shaffir, and Steven W. Kleinknecht. 2009. "Exercises in Reflexivity: Situating Theory in Practice." In *Ethnographies Revisited: Constructing Theory in the Field*, edited by Anthony J. Puddephatt, William Shaffir, and Steven W. Kleinknecht, 1–34. London, UK: Routledge.

Pullen, Lauren. 2015. "Interior Health Moving Forward with Laundry Privatization Proposal." *Global News*, 11 February. Accessed 29 February 2016.

http://globalnews.ca/news/1824597/interior-health-moving-forward-with-laundry-privatization-proposal/.

Ragone, Gina L. 2012. "Preventing Infection from Linens." *Long-Term Living* 61 (3): 29.

Rashid, Asaf. 2013. "Job Cuts in Laundry Services Hint at Larger Privatization Plan." *NB Media Co-op.* Accessed 17 April 2015. http://nbmediacoop .org/2013/11/04/job-cuts-to-laundry-workers-hint-at-a-larger-privatization-plan/.

Rolfe, Gary, Neil Jackson, Lyn Garner, Melanie Jasper, and Anne Gale. 1999. "Developing the Role of the Generic Healthcare Support Worker: Phase 1 of an Action Research Study." *International Journal of Nursing Studies* 36 (4): 323–34.

Romanow, Roy J. 2002. *Building on Values: The Future of Health Care in Canada. Commission on the Future of Health Care in Canada.* Ottawa: National Library of Canada.

Rosenberg, Harriet G. 1987. "The Kitchen and the Multinational Corporation: An Analysis of the Links between the Household and Global Corporations." *Journal of Business Ethics* 6:179–94.

Rosenthal, Carolyn, and Anne Martin-Matthews. 1999. "Families as Care Providers versus Care Managers? Gender and Type of Care in a Sample of Employed Canadians." SEDAP Research Paper No. 4. Hamilton: McMaster University.

Ross, Margaret M., Anne Carswell, and William Dalziel. 2001. "Family Caregiving in Long-Term Care Facilities." *Clinical Nursing Research* 10 (4): 347–63.

Sacouche, D.A., L.C. Morrone, and Joao Silvestre da Silva. 2012. "Impact of Ergonomics Risk among Workers in Clothes Central Distribution Service in a Hospital." *Work* 41 (1): 1836–40.

Saskatchewan Information and Privacy Commissioner. 2015. "Saskatchewan Information and Privacy Commissioner Review Report 082 2015." *Sunrise Regional Health Authority.* Accessed 1 July 2015. https://cupe.ca/sites/cupe/files/2015-07-17_final_report_082-2015.pdf.

Savishinsky, Joel S. 1991. *The Ends of Time: Life and Work in a Nursing Home.* New York: Bergin and Garvey.

Schensul, Stephen L., Jane J. Schensul and Margaret Diane LeCompte. 1999. *Essential Ethnographic Methods: Observations, Interviews and Questionnaires.* Walnut Creek, CA: Altamira Press.

Schnelle, John F., Sandra F. Simmons, Charlene Harrington, Mary Cadogan, Emily Garcia, and Barbara M. Bates-Jensen. 2004. "Relationship of Nursing

Home Staffing to Quality of Care." *Health Service Research* 39 (2): 225–50. doi:10.1111/j.1475-6773.2004.00225.x.

Scourfield, Peter. 2011. "Cartelization Revisited and the Lessons of Southern Cross." *Critical Social Policy* 32 (1): 137–48.

Sepkowitz, Kent A. 1996. "Occupationally Acquired Infections in Health Care Workers, Part II." *Annals of Internal Medicine* 125 (11): 917–28.

Shady, Kim. 2004. "Safety First for On-Premise Laundries." *Nursing Homes* 53 (8): 70–2.

– 2006. "An Ergonomic Look at Facility Laundry Rooms." *Nursing Homes* 55 (3): 88–9.

Sheth, Hitesh C. 2009. "Deinstitutionalization or Disowning Responsibility." *International Journal of Psychosocial Rehabilitation* 13 (2): 11–20.

Shiao, Judith S., M.L. McLaws, K.Y. Huang, and Yu-Liang Guo. 2001. "Sharps Injuries among Hospital Support Personnel." *Journal of Hospital Infection* 49 (4): 262–7.

Shultz, Erika. 2010. *The Long-Term Care System in Germany.* Berlin: Deutsches Institut für Wirtschtsforshunn.

Singh, Dara, G.J. Qadri, Monica Kotwal, A.T. Syed, and Farooq Jan. 2009. "Quality Control in Linen and Laundry Service at a Tertiary Care Teaching Hospital in India." *International Journal of Health Sciences* 3 (1): 33–44.

Sky, Laura. 1995. *Lean and Mean Health Care: The Creation of the Generic Worker and the Deregulation of Health Care.* Don Mills: The Ontario Federation of Labour.

Smith, Dorothy. 1987. *The Everyday World as Problematic.* Boston: Northeastern University Press.

Smith, Eileen. 2003. "Hidden Dangers." *Occupational Health* 55 (5), 27–9.

Standaert, Steven M., Robert H. Hutcheson, and William Schaffner. 1994. "Nosocomial Transmission of Salmonella Gastroenteritis to Laundry Workers in a Nursing Home." *Infection Control and Hospital Epidemiology* 15 (1): 22–6.

Stinson, Jane, Nancy Pollak, and Marcy Cohen. 2005. *The Pains of Privatization: How Contracting Out Hurts Health Support Workers, Their Families, and Health Care.* Canadian Centre for Policy Alternatives. Accessed 29 February 2016. http://www.policyalternatives.ca/sites/default/files/uploads/publications/BC_Office_Pubs/bc_2005/pains_priv_summary.pdf.

Stolt, Ragnar, Paula Blonquist, and Ulrika Winblas. 2011. "Privatization of Social Services: Quality Differences in Swedish Elderly Care." *Social Science & Medicine* 72 (4): 560–7.

Taft, Lois B., Kathleen Delaney, Dorothy Seman, and Jane Stansell. 1993. "Dementia Care: Creating a Therapeutic Milieu." *Journal of Gerontological Nursing* 19 (10): 30–9.

Tanuseputro, Peter, Mathieu Chalifoux, Carol Bennett, Andrea Gruneir, Susan E. Bronskill, Peter Walker, and Douglas Manuel. 2015. "Hospitalization and Mortality Rates in Long-Term Care Facilities: Does For-Profit Status Matter?" *Journal of the American Medical Directors Association* 16 (10): 874–83.

Tarbox, A.R. 1983. "The Elderly in Nursing Homes: Psychological Aspects of Neglect." *Clinical Gerontology* 1 (4): 39–52.

Texas Department of Insurance, Division of Worker Compensation and Workplace Safety. 2007. "Health Care Facilities and Workplace Violence Prevention." *Texas Department of Insurance.* Accessed 1 January 2016. http://www.tdi.texas.gov/pubs/videoresource/stpwpvhealthc.pdf.

Thielen, Belinda. 2003. "Laundry Workers: Cleaning Up an Industry." *Occupational Hazards*, October 2003.

Thompson, E.P. 1978. *The Poverty of Theory and Other Essays.* New York: Monthly Review Press.

Tice, Carol. 2014. "Best Franchises to Own: Why Home Healthcare Is Hot." *Forbes*, 27 May.

Tronto, Joan. 1993. *Moral Boundaries: A Political Argument for an Ethic of Care.* New York: Routledge.

Twigg, Julia. 2000. "Carework as a Form of Bodywork." *Ageing and Society* 20 (4): 389–411.

– 2002. "The Body in Social Policy: Mapping a Territory." *Journal of Social Policy* 31 (3): 421–39.

– 2007. "Clothing, Age and the Body: A Critical Review." *Ageing and Society* 27 (2): 285–305.

– 2010. "Clothing and Dementia: A Neglected Dimension?" *Journal of Aging Studies* 24 (4): 223–30.

Twigg, Julia, and Christina E. Buse. 2013. "Dress, Dementia and the Embodiment of Identity." *Dementia* 12 (3): 326–36.

Vabo, Mia, Karen Christensen, Frode Fadnes Jacobsen, and Håkon Dalby Trætteberg. 2013. "Marketisation in Norwegian Eldercare: Preconditions, Trends and Resistance." In *Marketization in Nordic Eldercare: A Research Report on Legislation, Oversight, Extent and Consequences*, edited by Gabrielle Meagher and Marta Szebehely, 163–202. Stockholm: Stockholm University.

Van de Walle, Steven, and Gerhard Hammerschmid. 2011. "The Impact of the New Public Management: Challenges for Coordination and Cohesion in European Public Sectors." *Halduskultuur – Administrative Culture* 12 (2): 190–209.

van Herk, Aritha. 2002. "Invisibled Laundry." *Signs* 27 (3): 893–900.

van Hoof, Joost, Helianthe S.M. Kort, H. van Waarde, and M.M. Blom. 2010. "Environmental Interventions and the Design of Homes for Older Adults with Dementia: An Overview." *American Journal of Alzheimer's Disease and Other Dementias* 25 (3): 202–32.

Vosko, Leah F. 2003. "The Pasts (and Futures) of Feminist Political Economy in Canada: Reviving the Debate." In *Studies in Political Economy: Developments in Feminism*, edited by Caroline Andrews, Pat Armstrong, Hugh Armstrong, Wallace Clement, and Leah F. Vosko, 305–32. Toronto: Women's Press.

– 2006. "Precarious Employment: Towards an Improved Understanding of Labour Market Insecurity." In *Precarious Employment: Understanding Labour Market Insecurity in Canada*, edited by Leah F. Vosko, 3–40. Montreal and Kingston: McGill-Queen's University Press.

Vosko, Leah F., and Mark Thomas. 2014. "Confronting the Employment Standards Enforcement Gap: Exploring the Potential for Union Engagement with Employment Law in Ontario, Canada." *Journal of Industrial Relations* 56 (5): 631–52.

Vrangbaek, Karsten, Ole Helby Petersen, and Olf Hjelmar. 2015. "Is Contracting Out Bad for Employees? A Review of International Experience." *Review of Public Personnel Administration* 35 (1): 3–23.

Wands, Susan E., and Annalee Yassi. 1993. "Modernization of a Laundry Processing Plant: Is It Really an Improvement?" *Applied Ergonomics* 24 (6): 387–96.

Ward, Richard, Antony A. Vass, Neeru Aggarwal, Cydonie Garfield, and Beau Cybyk. 2008. "A Different Story: Exploring Patterns of Communication in Residential Dementia Care." *Ageing and Society* 28 (5): 629–51.

Whiteside, Heather. 2015. *Purchase for Profit: Public-Private Partnerships and Canada's Public Health Care System*. Toronto: University of Toronto Press.

Wilkinson, Richard, and Michael Marmot. 1998. *Social Determinants of Health: The Solid Facts*. Geneva, Switzerland: World Health Organization, Centre for Urban Health.

Williamson, Julie E. 2011. "Awash in Productivity." *McKnight's Long-Term*

Care, 1 March. Accessed 29 February 2016. https://www.highbeam.com
/doc/1G1-259752393.html.

Witz, Anne. 1990. "Professions and Patriarchy: The Gendered Politics of
Occupational Closure." *Sociology* 24 (4): 675–90.

Wolcott, Harry F. 2008. *Ethnography: A Way of Seeing*. Lanham, Maryland:
AltaMira Press.

World Health Organization. 2010. "Classifying Health Workers: Mapping
Occupations to the International Standard Classification." *World Health
Organization*. Accessed 29 February 2016.
http://www.who.int/hrh/statistics/Health_workers_classification.pdf.

– 2012. "Country Profile of Occupational Health System in Germany."
World Health Organization. Accessed 29 February 2016. http://www.euro
.who.int/__data/assets/pdf_file/0010/178957/OSH-Profile-Germany.pdf.

Zimring, Randy. 1998. "Maximizing Laundry Productivity." *Nursing Homes
Long Term Care Management* 47 (9): 64–6.

Zuberi, Daniyal, and Melita B. Ptashnick. 2011. "The Deleterious Consequences of Privatization and Outsourcing for Hospital Support Work:
The Experiences of Contracted-Out Hospital Cleaners and Dietary Aids
in Vancouver, Canada." *Social Science and Medicine* 72 (6): 907–11.

Index